ॐ

Illustrated Samadhi Pada

The Science of Unlearning

Illustrations by Vishakha Rao

Dipanshu Aggarwal

Content copyright © Dipanshu Aggarwal 2023
Illustrations copyright © Vishakha Rao 2023

ISBN13: 978-93-95766-67-8 Paperback Edition
ISBN13: 978-93-95766-94-4 Hardbound Edition
ISBN13: 978-93-95766-79-1 Digital Edition

Title: **Illustrated Samadhi Pada**
SubTitle: **The Science of Unlearning**
Author: **Dipanshu Aggarwal**
Illustrator: **Vishakha Rao**

Dipanshu Aggarwal asserts the moral right to be identified as the author of this work.
All rights reserved. No part of this publication may be reproduced, stored in a retrieval system, or transmitted, in any form or by any means, mechanical, electronic, photocopying, recording or otherwise, without the prior permission of the publisher.

Printed and Published by
Devotees of Sri Sri Ravi Shankar Ashram
34 Sunny Enclave, Devigarh Road,
Patiala 147001, Punjab, Bhārat

https://advaita56.in/ The Art of Living Centre
https://www.arnavh.com/ Arnavh Yoga

Devotees Library Cataloging-in-Publication Data
Aggarwal, Dipanshu (Author). Rao, Vishakha (Illustrator).
Language: English. Thema: QDTM AKLB 2BBA 6CA
BISAC: OCC010000 BODY, MIND & SPIRIT / Mindfulness & Meditation
Keywords: 1. Patanjali Yoga Sutras. 2. Ashtanga Yoga. 3. Meditate. 4. Spiritual
Typeset in 12 YU Gothic UI

12th November 2023, Diwali
Kartik Masa, Krishna Paksha Chaturdashi Tithi, Swati Nakshatra
Hemant Ritu, Dakshinayana.
Vikram Samvat 2080 Pingala, Saka Era 1945 Shobhakrit

1st Edition November 2023

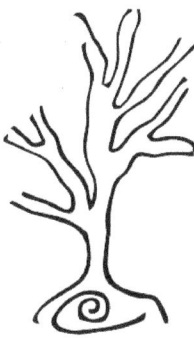

"From the solemn gloom of the temple children run out to play in the dust. God watches them play and forgets the priest."

- **Rabindranath Tagore**

ACKNOWLEDGEMENTS

I could write another book with just the names of people I should be acknowledging. I have been extremely lucky in the love and support I have received. Particularly, I express my heart-felt gratitude to my uncle Ashwini Kumar Aggarwal, whose energy, wisdom, and actions keep me motivated, to Jagjit Uncle whose every action inspires me, and to Willy Uncle, whose blessings do wonders beyond my imagination. Much love to Johann Arora for all the conversations. Cheers for my friends for the feedback, and the questions. Lastly, gratitude to the universe – for manifesting my desire to complete this book.

CREDITS

Nivas Hari Simha, B.Des – Visual Communication, Woxsen University, Hyderabad for illustrating five Sutras 1.1 to 1.5.

For my mother, whose courage surpasses all Knowledge.
For my Mammu, whose patience humbles Death.
For my sister, whose hope makes magic.
For my grandfather, whose resilience breaks mountains.
.
For my friend, who gives me hope.

PREVIOUS WORK BY THE SAME AUTHOR

84 Yoga Asanas Fitness Postures
https://www.amazon.com/dp/B09CV558XV/

YOGA Surya Namaskar
https://www.amazon.com/dp/B08C7Y7L48/

Gheranda Samhita the foundation of Modern Yoga
https://www.amazon.com/dp/B08WYXTKQ8/

Live One Hour Yoga Sessions
https://www.amazon.com/dp/B0BPYM6DX6/

Arnavh Yoga
https://www.amazon.com/dp/B0BYXH3PVR/

Tough Stance Strength Flexibility Alertness
https://www.amazon.com/dp/B09JN5PL2Y/

Egypt – Going Back In Time
https://www.amazon.com/dp/B078VDKCSJ/

FOREWORD

I have known Dipanshu since the beginning of my Yoga training Journey. Even then Dipanshu was already a well read 'yogi,' deeply connected to the yoga philosophy. His sincerity towards the subject and his deep thinking has always kept me in awe. As yoga teachers our conversations have revolved around Yoga, spirituality, our experiences with Yoga techniques, and the knowledge of ancient literatures. His depth of all these topics is seen in this book. The way he has always cleared my doubts about techniques in such clear, simple manner always kept me interested in listening to his views of yoga subjects.

This book is a must read for anyone who wants to take responsibility of their personal and spiritual growth in life. Whichever background you are from, this book will contribute to your growth. It interprets the ancient wisdom of mind management and the ways to make your mind your friend. The detailed interpretation of the 'Sutras' are in a manner which can be understood by anyone, whether one is from the yoga community or not. The examples and experiences mentioned to explain the points are relatable and are made practical so that we can make it a part of our day-to-day life.

Currently, the world has the highest percentage of people suffering from mental stress. Psychosomatic diseases are becoming common and talked about. Books like these give us a pathway to overcome and deal with them.

The book is simple, precise, and yet profound which can be relatable for a person of any age. The graphics and quotes used in the book keeps the reader involved. Dipanshu's keen interest in the subject of yoga, his experience of teaching and his motivation to go deep into a subject philosophy is notable in this book.

I wish the readers can experience this journey of inner exploration through this book.

JOHANN ARORA
MSc. Yoga Therapy, SVYASA

SANSKRIT TO ENGLISH TRANSLITERATION GUIDE

अ a pronounced like 'a' in Alone

आ (ा) ā pronounced like 'a' in Arm

इ (ि) i pronounced like 'i' in Sit

ई (ी) ī pronounced like 'ee' in Steep

उ (ु) u pronounced like 'u' in Put

ऊ (ू) ū pronounced like 'oo' in Tool

ए (े) e pronounced like 'ay' in Day

ऐ (ै) ai pronounced like 'ai' in Aisle

ओ (ो) o pronounced like 'o' in Flow

औ (ौ) au pronounced like 'ow' in Owl

ḥ (ः) soft echo of the preceding alphabet

क (ka) — wick
ख (kha) — Khyber
ग (ga) — grab
घ (gha) — ghost
ङ (ṅa) — ink
च (ca) — chat
ज (ja) — jam
छ (cha) — touch hue
झ (jha) — taj hue
ञ (ña) — inch

ट (ṭa) — tablet
ठ (ṭha) — Vithal
ड (ḍa) — deer
ढ (ḍha) — good hue
ण (ṇ) — onion
त (ta) — pasta
थ (tha) — thought
द (da) — that
ध (dha) — M.S Dhoni
न (na) — never

प (pa) — pink
फ (ph) — fever
ब (ba) — best
भ (bha) — abhor
म (ma) — mask
य (ya) — yesterday
र (ra) — rinse
ळ (la) — land
व (va) — vase

श (śa) — shine
ष (ṣa) — leash
स (sa) — solid
ह (ha) — hat

त्र (Tra) — tram (with soft t as in pasta)
क्ष (kṣa) — rickshaw
श्र (śra) — shriek

Many sounds of the Devanagari script do not exist in the English language. These alphabets and the corresponding English words which come close to the actual pronunciation are given below.

छ (cha) — tou<u>ch h</u>ue
झ (jha) — ta<u>j h</u>ue
ढ (ḍha) — goo<u>d h</u>ue
ण (ṇ) — onion
ज्ञ (jña) — i<u>gn</u>oble

TABLE OF CONTENTS

FOREWORD 6

SANSKRIT TO ENGLISH TRANSLITERATION GUIDE 9

PRAYER 15

INTRODUCTION 17

1.1 THE TIME IS NOW 21

1.2 REIGNING IN THE MIND 25

1.3 COMING HOME 27

1.4 THE BOURNE IDENTITY 29

1.5 UNDER THE UMBRELLA 31

1.6 THE FAMOUS FIVE 33

1.7 PROOF AND BEYOND 37

1.8 THE GREAT HOUDINI 41

1.9 ALL IS IN WONDERLAND 45

1.10 SLEEPY HEAD 51

1.11 DON'T YOU REMEMBER? 53

1.12 THE TWIN TOWERS	57
1.13 THE PRACTICE OF PRACTICE	59
1.14 THE NATURE OF PRACTICE	63
1.15 THE PARADOX OF DETACHMENT	67
1.16 TRANSCENDING TRINITY	71
1.17 HALF-AWAKE	75
1.18 HALF-ASLEEP	79
1.19 DISSOLVE	83
1.20 SOWING SEEDS	87
1.21 A CALL TO THE UNIVERSE	91
1.22 MORE SUGAR MORE SWEETNESS	93
1.23 TRUMP CARD	97
1.24 THE GOD PARTICLE	101
1.25 THE THEORY OF EVERYTHING	105
1.26 THE MASTER	107
1.27 SOUND OF GOD	109
1.28 THE SECRET OF MANTRA	113

1.29 **THE POWER OF MANTRA**   **115**

1.30 **THE CHALLENGE**   **117**

1.31 **WATCH OUT FOR THE SIGNS**   **123**

1.32 **ONE THING TO RULE THEM ALL**   **127**

1.33 **PEOPLE PEOPLE EVERYWHERE**   **131**

1.34 **MIND YOUR BREATH**   **137**

1.35 **THE REAL-SURREAL CONNECTIONS**   **141**

1.36 **THERE IS A LIGHT THAT NEVER GOES OUT**   **143**

1.37 **BE LIKE WATER MY FRIEND**   **147**

1.38 **WIDE ASLEEP**   **151**

1.39 **AS YOU LIKE IT**   **157**

1.40 **WORLD IN THE PALM OF MY HAND**   **161**

1.41 **ETERNAL SUNSHINE OF THE SPOTLESS MIND**   **165**

1.42 **WHAT'S IN A NAME?**   **171**

1.43 **EMPTINESS**   **175**

1.44 **CHEWING GUM**   **179**

1.45 **BRUCE ALMIGHTY**   **183**

[1.46](#) **THE SEED OF EXISTENCE**   **187**

[1.47](#) **I AM THAT**   **189**

[1.48](#) **THE ABSOLUTE**   **191**

[1.49](#) **BREAKING DAWN**   **193**

[1.50](#) **THE SEED OF CREATION**   **195**

[1.51](#) **I AM**   **197**

EPILOGUE   **199**

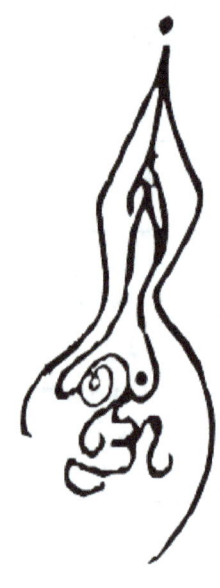

PRAYER

योगेन चित्तस्य पदेन वाचां मलं शरीरस्य च वैद्यकेन ।
योऽपाकरोत्तं प्रवरं मुनीनां पतञ्जलिं प्राञ्जलिरानतोऽस्मि ॥

yogena cittasya padena vācāṃ malaṃ śarīrasya ca vaidyakena l
yo'pākarottaṃ pravaraṃ munīnāṃ patañjaliṃ prāñjalirānato'smi ll

By Yogic practice the purity of the Mind,
by Grammar sweetness of the Tongue,
by Ayurveda who banished illness of the Bodily,
to that revered sage PATANJALI
who made it all happen, my sincerest salutation.

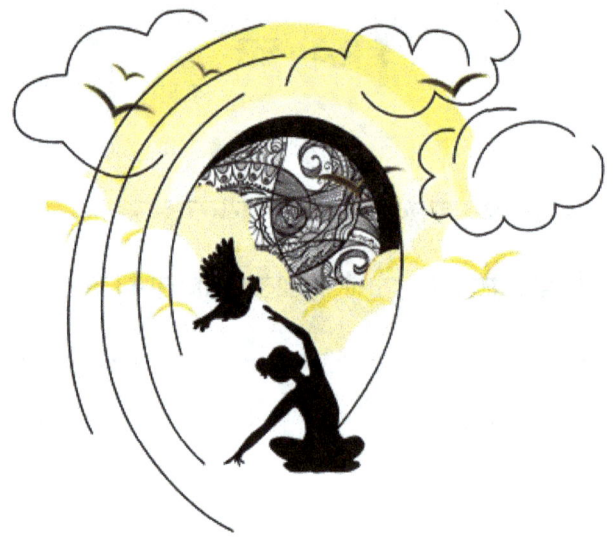

INTRODUCTION

We spend a lot of life looking for answers. Our life looms over us like a big question, never letting us rest, never letting us stop. There is no end to the things we do for those answers. We go around the world, we climb mountains, we dive into the seas, and we sing songs to the moon. There is no end, except for one little thing. We never turn in. We never stop to seek answers in our own self. We never seek to scale the walls our minds create. No one can give us any answers. We enjoy listening to many philosophers and saints, we intellectualize the knowledge they give in their infinite compassion, but even then, the purpose of the knowledge is not to provide answers. If answers could be found just by listening or reading a book, the entire world would have become enlightened a long time ago.

The purpose of knowledge is simple – it motivates us to find our own answers. It plants a seed of curiosity – we start asking the big questions. Once the questions are right, and the intent to look for answers is unshakeable, the answers reveal themselves. It is inevitable. Truth cannot be denied to those who seek it.

Keeping this fundamental, irrevocable principle in mind, let us move forward in this journey towards understanding Maharishi Patanjali.

Samadhi Pada

Yoga Sutras of Patanjali

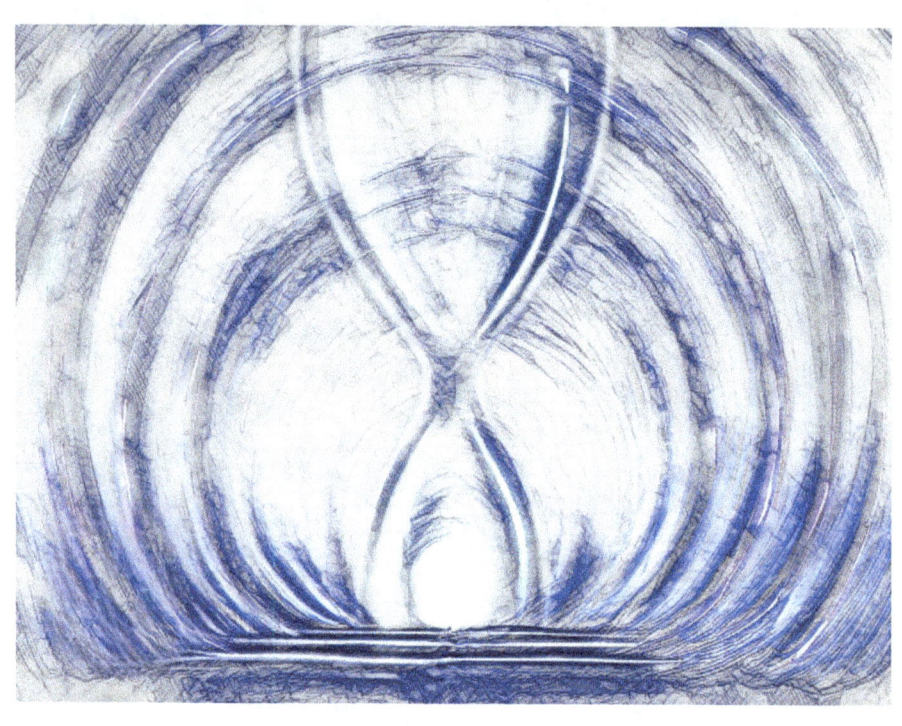

1.1

THE TIME IS NOW

अथ योगानुशासनम् ॥
atha yogānuśāsanam ॥
(Atha Yoga Anushasanam)

Now, I enunciate the discipline of Yoga.

"Generally speaking, now is as good a time as any."
- Hugh Laurie

NOW. Is there anything beyond Now? Inhalation is Now, exhalation is Now. Past is Now, future is Now. Creation is Now, dissolution is Now. Life is Now, and Death is now. I am Now. You are Now. Liberation is Now. Nothing is Now. Everything is Now.

The past has gone by, and yet the mind clings to it like a parasite. The future is yet to come, and the mind wants to live it beforehand. It has done this for a long time, for lifetimes. One day, blessedly, it gets tired. It comes to rest. The mind turns inwards. There is a light. It becomes unattached to that is without and starts attuning itself to what is within. There is so much that has been accumulated – trash kept in vaults. There is pleasure, pain, love, hate, jealousy, and resentment. There is pride of wealth, and burden of the roles it has played. But what is it? What is it without the things that have been accumulated? This is when one is humble and ready to listen to knowledge of the Self.

It is a perilous task, this quest to know "Who am I?" It is not for the weak. It requires courage, and faith. It requires commitment. The road is long and tricky, and obstacles abound at each bend. Only discipline will see the journey through to completion.

Since childhood, the word discipline has meant constriction, a lack of freedom, and suppression – one that teachers would scream all day long to suppress our play and laughter in the classrooms. Even now, when I hear the word, my gut twists a little in apprehension. *What tyranny am I going to be subjected to?* How can constriction lead to expansion? How can suppression lead to wholeness? How can finite lead to infinite?

The mind is a tricky customer, a mischievous monkey that keeps jumping from one tree to another, taking a bite out of one fruit after the other, and pulling the tails of other animals because it is fun. The mind enjoys sensory pleasures, but is not able to experience any true joy, for it is too scattered, too occupied with what was and what will be. Such a mind cannot, but end up falling into suffering and misery.

Discipline is needed to focus the mind when one is doing something that may not be a pleasant experience but will result in a fruit that is desirable and joyful. Discipline is the key to accomplish anything, for discipline encompasses commitment, determination and will power. Discipline is needed when one needs to study for 10 hours a day for 6-8 months and clear an important exam. Discipline is needed to meet deadlines by giving up leisure time. Discipline is needed to follow an exercise routine. Discipline is required even to do things that one enjoys but is irregular with.

Discipline is not freedom – it earns freedom. Discipline is not infinite – it earns the infinite. The discipline required to answer the query "Who am I?" cannot be imposed from outside. Such desire must burn within, and discipline must be self-imposed to keep moving. This self-imposed discipline is Yoga.

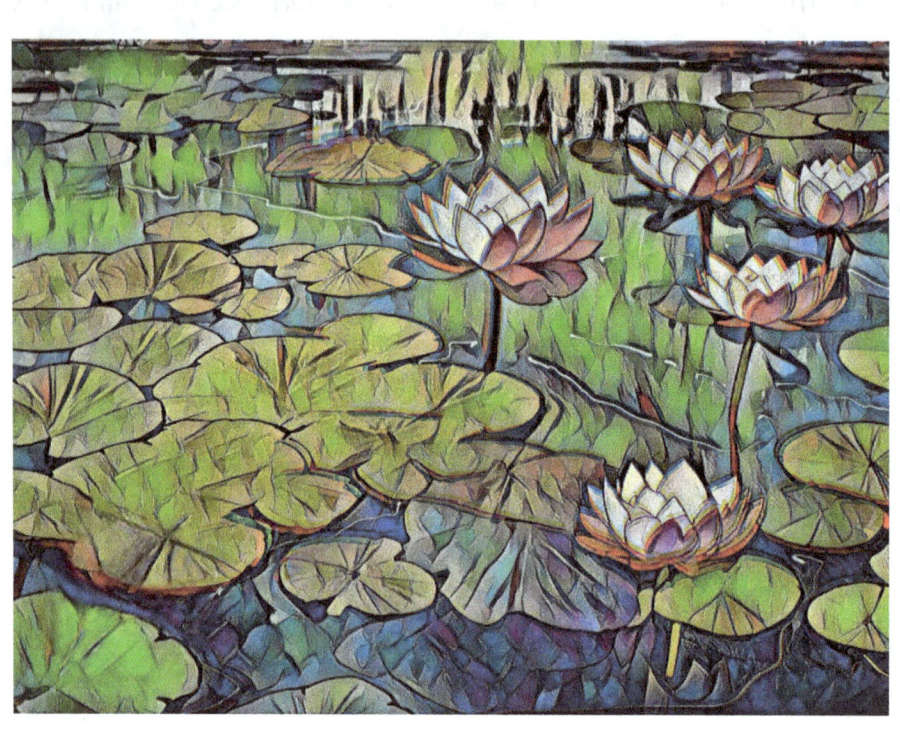

1.2

REIGNING IN THE MIND

योगश्चित्तवृत्तिनिरोधः ॥
yogaścittavṛttinirodhaḥ ||
(Yoga Chitta Vritti Nirodha)

To block the circular patterns of consciousness is Yoga.

"When the mind is kept away from its preoccupation, it becomes quiet."
-Nisargadatta Maharaj

Chitta means 'to be conscious of.' It represents the entire spectrum of consciousness which includes the intellect, memory, ego, and the mind in which thoughts arise.

The consciousness is the sky, pure and always untainted. Vrittis are like the clouds - the modifications/modulations happening in the consciousness. The thoughts and desires, dreams and actions, ambitions and fears, awareness and sleep, convictions and doubts, likes and dislikes, are all modulations of the consciousness – different clouds that that arise in the sky. The Vrittis keep on churning the consciousness, and awareness stays on the surface. If it stays on surface for a long time, it forgets its own depth. All these processes of Chitta start covering the consciousness as impressions and the consciousness starts to identify itself as each individual cloud, forgetting itself to be the sky in which the clouds arise and dissolve. This brings about the limited scope of mind, breeding ego. It results in Karma - action done with sense of doership, the desire of whose fruit itself is another impression and results in manifestation of events which demands more action, and the cycle continues.

Nirodhah means to block or subdue. Yoga is not blocking the consciousness, but rather blocking/subduing the patterns of the consciousness that keep on following each other in an endless circle. The consciousness is never resting when the patterns are flowing. Suppression is not the aim here. Yoga is taking control of Chitta so that one has the discipline to be unaffected by the wavering desires and thoughts that keep on arising, and again rest in Silence.

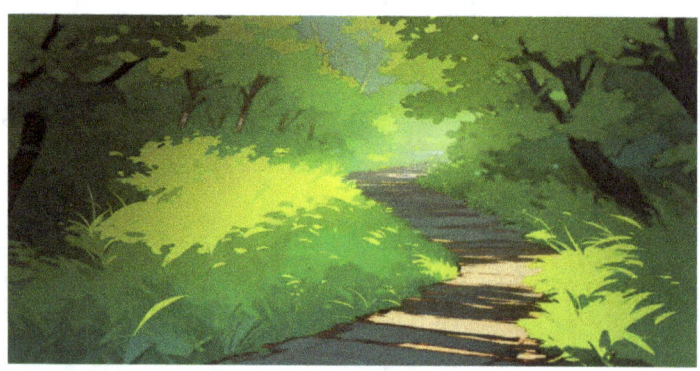

1.3

COMING HOME

तदा द्रष्टुः स्वरूपेऽवस्थानम् ॥
tadā draṣṭuḥ svarūpe'vasthānam ॥
(Tada Drashtu Svarupe Avasthanam)

Then the Seer (the Being) gets established in its true nature.

"There is no spoon."
- The Matrix

Once the vrittis are subdued, the consciousness relaxes and takes a step back, and assumes the role of the witness. This witness conscious cannot be achieved by *doing*, but by *being*. To simply be, in the act of non-doing reveals this state. Then, a state of lasting peace, focus and joy dawns. Then, one can access the vrittis as a tool. The knowledge of the vrittis is more academic than spiritual. At different stages of life, different vrittis will arise (and should arise). Ambition is important at a young age to earn success and achievements. Pride builds character. There will be desires that must be fulfilled, otherwise the mind will not settle down in any activity. However, having the skill to detach from the desires, the knowledge to use the mind as a tool, and the experience of the fulfilment that resides within, one passes through life like a cloud – living in the world, but staying untouched. The knowledge of the vrittis is for the scholars who wish to discuss and debate the Yoga Sutras of Patanjali and are not experiencing Yoga.

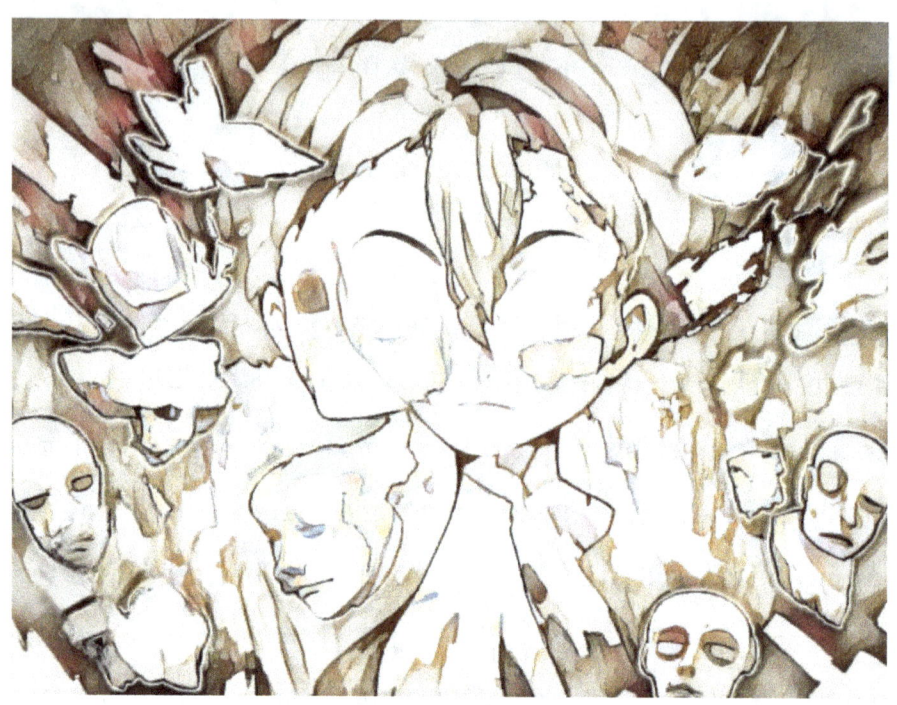

1.4

THE BOURNE IDENTITY

वृत्तिसारूप्यमितरत्र ॥
vṛttisārūpyamitaratra ॥
(Vritti Sarupyam Itaratra)

One identifies himself with the modulations of the mind.

"Play with your identifications – don't let them rule you."
-Sadhguru

Have you ever sat down with an emotion? Not acting on it, not wishing it to change, not distracting yourself. Where do you feel your anger in your body? Where do you feel love? Where does the loneliness make you feel empty? Where does the fear hold you hostage?

We have never learnt to observe our emotions – when we get angry, we flow in anger. We shout, or throw things around. Or, we suppress the outburst, letting the anger burn in our blood. When we are happy, even then we lose our sense of being. We become insensitive - we do not realise sometimes what we are doing or saying. When we watch an interesting movie, we lose all sense of the body and mind; we cry, we laugh and fall in love along with the characters. There is a magical quality of emotions; they sneak up on us, and before we know it, we have been hijacked. We do not feel, nay, we *become* the emotion.

It takes only a few years after we are born for us to start defining ourselves as the thoughts we have; when someone asks us about ourselves, we tell them what we like and dislike. Our preferences, and our experiences *become* us. We stop acting certain ways, because *that is not who I am*. We do things because that is what is expected of us. We are locked in a box of people's opinion and our ideas about ourselves. The desires cloud our judgement and intellect. Our identity becomes founded on a wisp of smoke. Where is the autonomy? Where is the free will? The potential and vastness of our existence is reduced to a few thoughts and emotions.

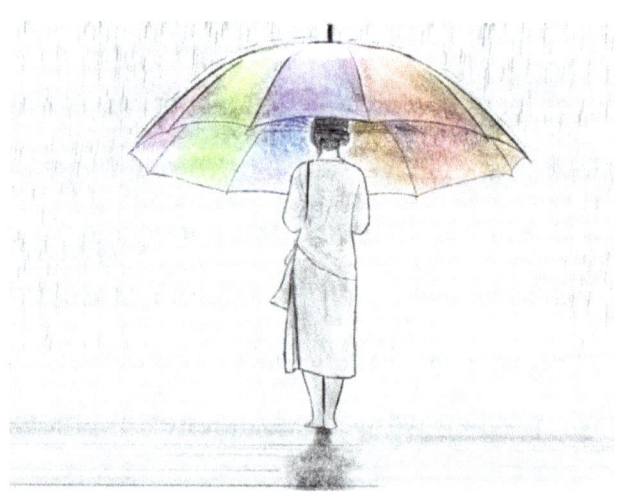

1.5

UNDER THE UMBRELLA

वृत्तयः पञ्चतय्यः क्लिष्टाक्लिष्टाः ॥
vṛttayaḥ pañcatayyaḥ kliṣṭākliṣṭāḥ ॥
(Vrittya Panchatya Klishta Aklishta)

The modifications of the mind are of five types; they can be pleasant or unpleasant.

"Like our stomachs, our minds are hurt more often by overeating than by hunger." -Petrarch

The modes in which the mind can function are very limited, in fact there are only 5 in number. Nonetheless, there is a great capacity for numerous thoughts to arise. While, to the unaware the thoughts may seem novel, they seldom are. Out of the thousands and thousands of thoughts, there is rarely a new thought. New ideas and thoughts require space which is available only in expanded awareness. In the current age of "hustling," there is no time to sit and stare out a window. Doing nothing is absolutely a terrifying idea.

The modes of the mind are five in number – there are no thoughts that cannot be categorised under one of these.

Depending on the situation, the mode of the mind may give rise either to a pleasant thought or an unpleasant thought.

For a few people only may this information serve any kind of purpose of advancing on the path of Yoga. Practicing awareness of the type of vrittis manifesting in the mind may help the practitioner assume an observer's seat.

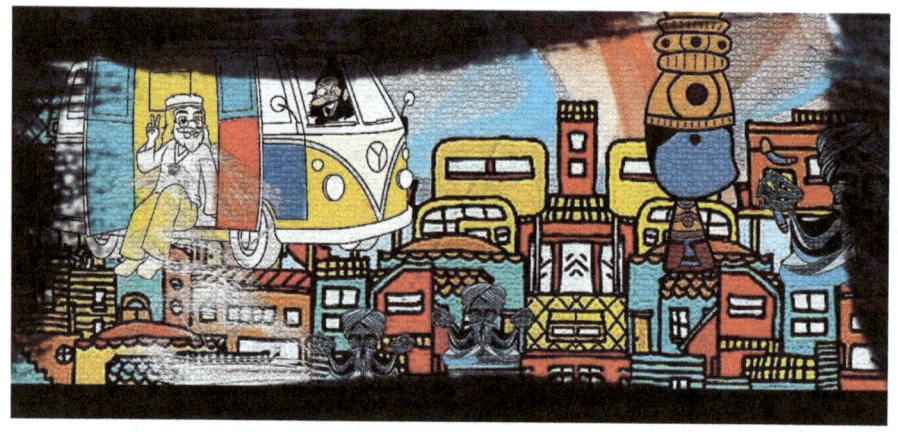

1.6

THE FAMOUS FIVE

प्रमाणविपर्ययविकल्पनिद्रास्मृत्यः ॥
pramāṇaviparyayavikalpanidrāsmṛtayaḥ ॥
(Pramana-Viparyaya-Vikalpa-Nidra-Smriti)

The five categories of the modulations of the mind are – Evident, Erroneous, Fanciful, Sleep and Reminiscence.

> "To go within one must first understand the principal thing, which is to be terribly honest to oneself, so that there is no deception whatsoever."
> - J. Krishnamurti

Every observation must take into account the observer. The act of observation itself alters that which is observed, hence we do not know the nature of that which is observed beyond our observation. The state of the mind of the person is one of the primary factors. A big festival in an exotic land with good music, abundant food and drink, and friendly people can also be described as "nonsensical tradition in a strange foreign land which gives an excuse to create noise pollution, and waste food and drink." One scenery but two completely opposite perspectives. Even the same person can experience the same situation in different ways. It is both a blessing and a curse. A familiar situation while bringing a sense of novelty, never quite meets our expectations. It is not the event, but how we respond to the event that forms our experience. The experience continues to affect our further decisions that consequently affect future experiences. All our thoughts that arise corresponding to every situation and event in our life are not descriptive of the nature of the event but of the state of the mind at the particular moment. This is why our experience of an event can even change after the event has passed if we get more information. The brain interprets and analyses; it does not simply see what is there. If we become familiar with this process and observe it from a distance, we can relieve the mind of its concepts and impressions and make effort to see each moment as it is, effectively living in the present moment.

The five categories under which all the Vrittis of the consciousness can be categorized are:

1. Pramana – proof. The inclination to look for evidence is Pramana Vritti. It includes knowledge gained by accumulating evidence.
2. Viparyaya – wrong knowledge. The inclination to assume things due to emotional instability. It results in knowledge obtained by error in judgement/perception. Once Viparyaya dawns, there is no space in the mind for Pramana.
3. Vikalpa – fanciful thoughts. All phobias, daydreams, anxieties, and hallucinations fall under the category of Vikalpa.
4. Nidra – sleep.
5. Smriti – Memory. It includes conscious, subconscious, and unconscious memory, not just stored in the mind, but memory stored in the body as well.

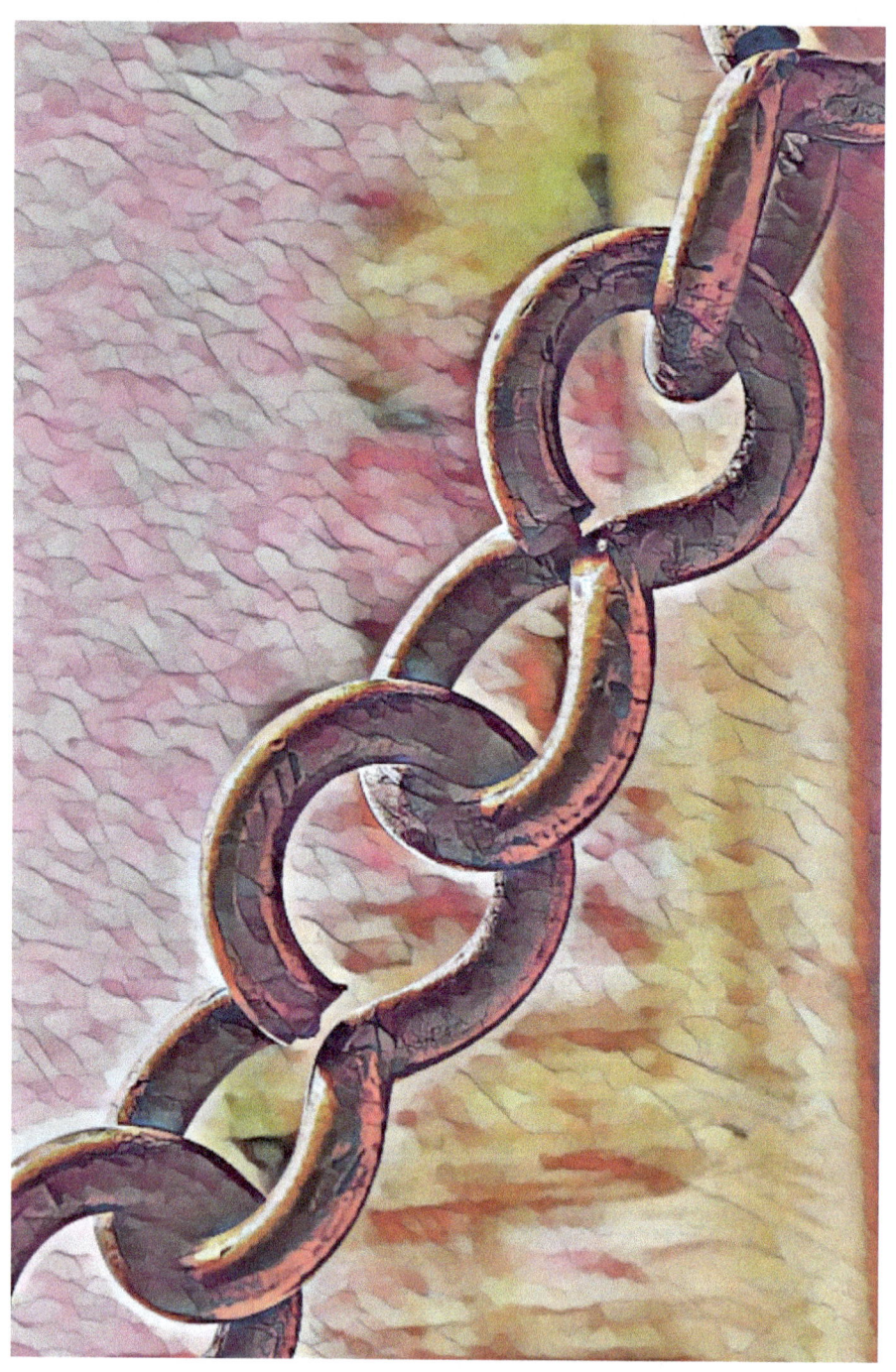

1.7

PROOF AND BEYOND

प्रत्यक्षानुमानागमाः प्रमाणानि ॥
pratyakṣānumānāgamāḥ pramāṇāni ॥
(Pratyakasha Anumana Agama Pramanani)

Evidence based cognition, inference and testimony are the sources of Pramana.

"A mind all logic is like a knife all blade. It makes the hand bleed that uses it." - Rabindranath Tagore

Maharishi Patanjali gives the three sources of information/knowledge through which the mind manifests in Pramana Vritti – or Right Knowledge.

The first source of Pramana is Pratyaksha - knowledge which is obtained by direct cognition – one sees a flower and smells it; it is a proof that the flower has some fragrance. We hear a child crying and see a crying child in front of us, it is proof of why we heard crying. When we wake up in the morning, the first thing we do is look for proof that we are in the same place where we fell asleep. However, even direct cognition does not ensure that the knowledge obtained is error-free. We all have experience mirages. Just because it can be seen, does not mean its real. On the other hand, just because it cannot be cognized by our limited senses, does not validate its absence. Absence of proof is not proof of absence.

The second source of Pramana is inference – Anumana. The knowledge thus obtained is based on reasoning and experience. The knowledge is right knowledge or Pramana if it based on sound reasoning. A person happily jumping while watching a sports match can correctly cause someone to infer his preferred team is winning the match – our years of experience of our own behavior in such situations has given us experience. We guess the breakfast by the smell wafting around the house, or that mother is in a foul mood because she uncharacteristically quiet, and has a scary frown on her face. Experience and sound reasoning provide us with clues to navigate our life. We spend a lot of time in this vritti – we try to guess why someone said so and so to us, why someone acts the way we do and try to put labels on personalities and try to come with theories to explain events from very limited information.

The last source of Pramana is collective knowledge, or something that has been written. Traditionally it meant the knowledge contained the ancient scriptures, or the testimony of a very learned person who surely has right knowledge. Such testimony could provide the right knowledge even if the person receiving it has not directly perceived it, and has no hints to infer it. The knowledge of Vedas, Upanishads, Bhagavad Gita is said to be infallible because it has been perceived in higher states of consciousness. Fundamentally, Agama means that which is believed by a lot of people. Today, WhatsApp messages, Facebook posts and Twitter comments are Agama. People blindly believe what is written there about unaware citizens, celebrities, and politicians. Death hoaxes, false cancer fundraisers, and celebrity scandals make the rounds and are talk of class rooms and office lunch tables. There is no proof of these news items except that it has been found in collective knowledge. One is not afraid to be a fool when there are a thousand fools to stand with. It has become so ingrained in our habits, that we have lost the ability to form personal opinions. We even like or dislike YouTube videos based on the comments of other people. Therefore, even Agama needs to be reliable for it to be right knowledge. The mind manifests solidly with some proof, otherwise it is shaky. In our day-to-day life, there are a lot of instances when Pramana Vritti is necessary, even necessary for survival. It is not to be understood that this category of thought process should be done away with. However, letting proof limit our awareness robs us of a fulfilling experience of life.

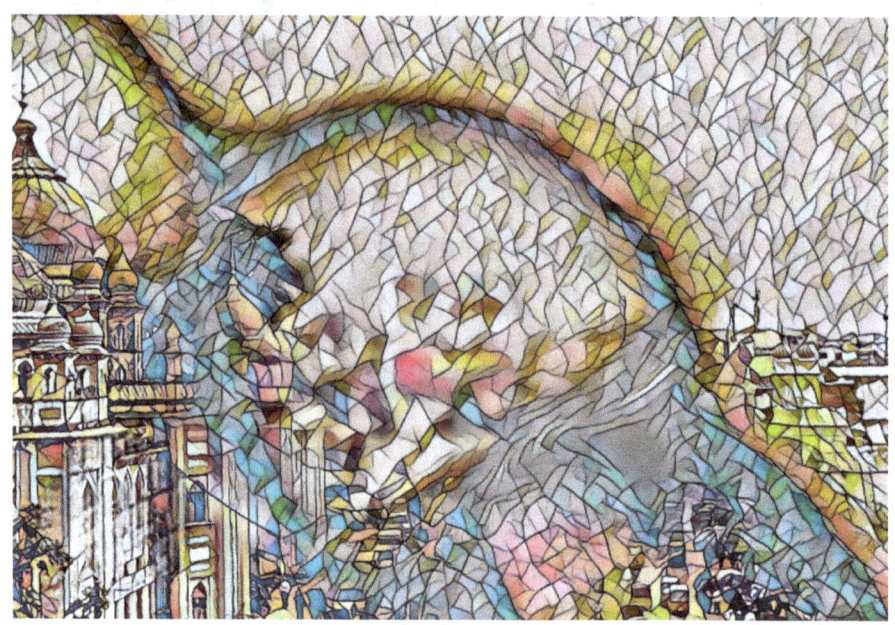

1.8

THE GREAT HOUDINI

विपर्ययो मिथ्याज्ञानमतद्रूपप्रतिष्ठम् ॥
viparyayo mithyājñānamatadrūpapratiṣṭham ॥
(Viparyaya Mithya Gyanam atadrupa pratishtham)

Misconceptions (Viparyaya) are false knowledge based on wrong perception.

"Opinion is the really the lowest form of human knowledge."
- Bill Bullard

Viparyaya is the second modulation of the mind. Viparyaya is erroneous knowledge, obtained due to bias, prejudice, moodiness, food, environment, time, or simply limited awareness. Here the correct form (the concept) is not grasped by the perceiver and that which is not there is perceived – hence it is called *atadrupapratishtham*.

In the modern age it has become very common to live in Viparyaya due to extensive use of virtual modes of communication. Instagram photos give the idea that the other person is living a very care-free life. Many people post edited photos using exotic locations and luxurious resorts – these people suffer through the misconception that envy of others shall be fulfilling or maybe delude themselves into becoming happy with the adulation rather than working hard on transforming the fantasy into truth.

News channels are one of the main reasons most of the people build concepts that have nothing to do with reality. The structure of such channels is such that one starts believing that everyone is out to do evil things only for personal gain and there is no room for kindness and compassion in this world. We start teaching children not to be cautious but to be suspicious and distrustful of everyone they meet. We start doubting our own family and friends who have been life-long pillars and have nourished us selflessly. The idea of romanticising a tragedy has also become another pandemic that is causing a lot of imagined distress. Emotions and imagination take hold of the mind and it starts believing in concepts that have no connection of what really is.

But we all have experienced some particular events when we dropped all logic and rationalism in frustration and rolled with emotions. Someone says "No" to you when you ask them for help after you had had a very exhausting day, and your frustrated mind makes you believe that they are out to pull you down. Someone may have always operated under self-doubt and low self-esteem and they will find that the person in front of them is not giving them enough attention and think of the other person as self-centered and arrogant.

When wrong knowledge gets established, no proof or logic stands. At that time, the vritti of Pramana (discussed in the previous sutra) is desirable and shall act as a tool to dissipate the clouds of Viparyaya. Most of the time, we impose our own emotions of what should be and should not be, concepts of right and wrong upon situations and people, thus, disallowing ourselves to be open to receive what really is. Somewhere deep down, the rational part of the mind tries to bring clarity, but it needs awareness to let it guide us. Subduing this vritti is important to keep it away from falling into traps.

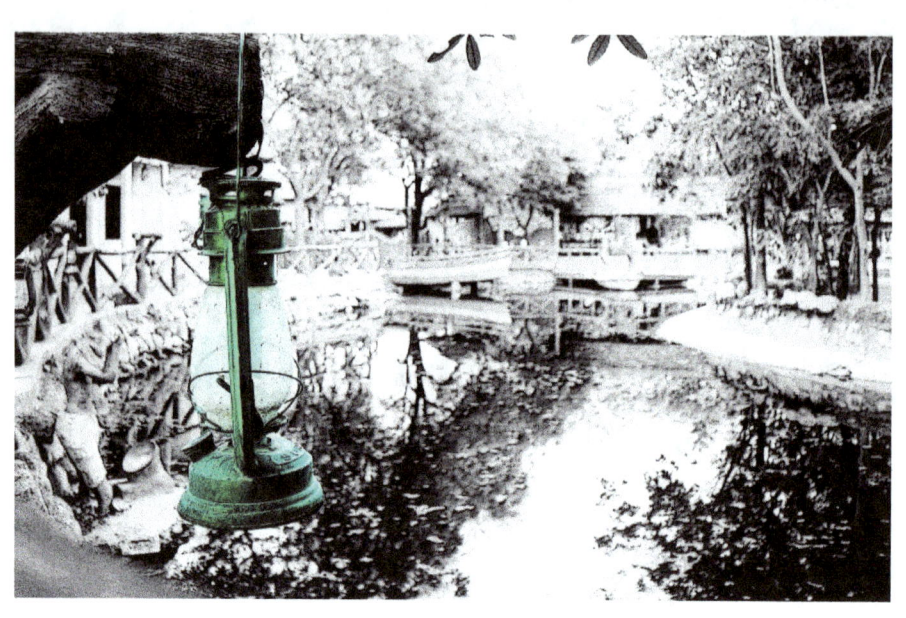

1.9

ALL IS IN WONDERLAND

शब्दज्ञानानुपाती वस्तुशून्यो विकल्पः ॥
śabdajñānānupātī vastuśūnyo vikalpaḥ ॥
(Shabda Gyana anupati Vastu-shunya Vikalpa)

Knowledge that is founded only on words, and has no real object; is Fantasy.

"Fear kills more dreams than failure ever will."
-Suzy Kassem

How many dreams have succumbed to fear, doubt, and inaction? How many lives have ended unfulfilled? How many potentials never realised? Things have never been this convenient before. Yet, somehow, while the world has shrunk and become closer, it has become increasingly difficult to navigate. Maybe it has shrunk so much, there is no space left to breathe.

We are living in our heads. We want to be prepared for the next second. We want to be prepared for the next day. We want to be prepared for the next 10 years. While preparing for a life, we have forgotten to live. We have become so conditioned to be prepared for everything, that we do not even want to leave a little corner for unpredictability in our lives. How can we then expect magic to happen?

We keep working out scenarios. Reality cannot be captured by our limited faculties of rationality and logic. *What if this happens, what if that happens...what if they laugh at me...what if I am not enough...?* How many times have a situation turned out exactly the way you thought it would? Never.

In recent times, "psychosomatic diseases" has become a common term in the world of medical science which is fortunate, and also sad. Many major diseases involving the heart, kidneys, and other major organs, and especially neurological disorders are psychosomatic in a large portion of patients. We as a society are currently overwhelmed by information, most of which is either untrue, insignificant, or irrelevant. The brain has an infinite capacity to hold information, and the mind has the annoying habit of bringing up these bits of information without cause -

this has resulted in a lot of stress, anxiety, and nervous tension for so many people because the mind just won't stop chattering. Neurological disorders seep down into the Pranic body causing blockages in the psychic channels (the Nadis) which carry the vital energy to each cell of the body. As a final result, the physical body becomes diseased.

All the phobias, paranoia, and hallucinations are different dimensions of Vikalpa. Phobias and other mental states which detach a person from a reality may stem from deep-rooted trauma or experiences and impressions in the mind that disrupted the normal functioning of the mind. It is possible that some of these impressions may be of the past lives. It is not under control for most of people suffering from such disorders and they need to be helped in every way possible. It has also been observed in modern psychological therapies that becoming aware of the impressions in the subconscious that are causing such fears and accepting them can reduce the fears and, in some cases, eliminate the manifestations completely.

Even on the spiritual path, it is common for practitioners to get stuck in Vikalpa. They imagine unprecedent outcomes – some of the most common desires among spiritual practitioners are: "I will never be in an undesirable state of mind", "I will never be afraid of any challenge that life may throw at me", "I will never get upset with anyone", "I will never live a day in poor health", etc. Change and decay are the nature of the mind-body complex and it is nothing wrong in getting upset or sad; the knowledge teaches that these are all temporary states and must not be allowed to drive our actions, and it provides us with the tools and the techniques to overcome bad days.

On the other side, Vikalpa may come in handy in many situations. Creating fanciful scenarios are beneficial in the creative field, especially for writers. Creating something is invaluable and if Vikalpa is the means to do so for a person, then so be it. But it must be followed by effort in present time for something to be created. Vikalpa is a very important process of the mind that can be fulfilling but like all other things, there must be a balance. No matter what, one must not lose touch with the reality.

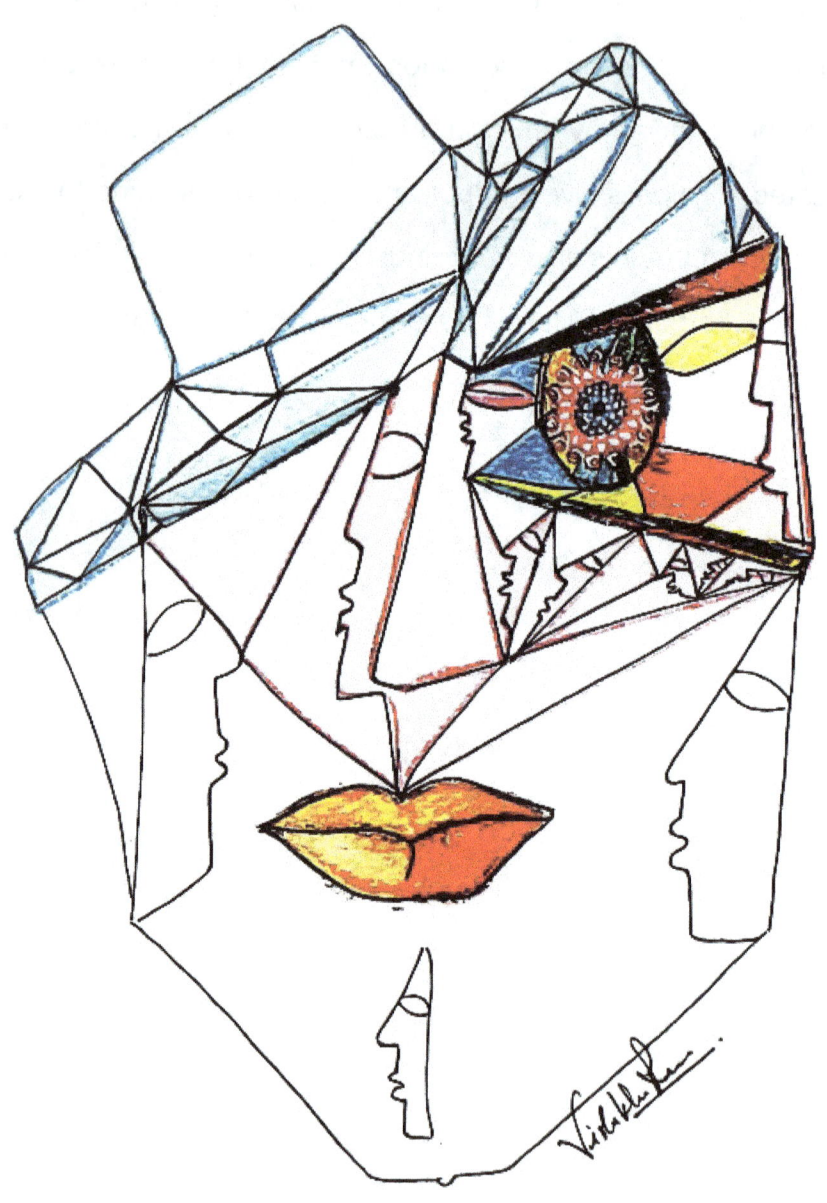

1.10

SLEEPY HEAD

अभावप्रत्ययालम्बना वृत्तिर्निद्रा ॥
abhāvapratyayālambanā vṛttirnidrā ॥
(Abhava pratyaya-alambana vritti Nidra)

The absence of any content upon which mind can support itself; is the state of Sleep.

"Be at rest. Be at peace. May the stars watch over you tonight." - Dipanshu Aggarwal

All the three Vrittis earlier discussed processed some idea or information or idea in the mind. The mind was conscious. When the mind is not in of the previous three states, it can be in Sleep or Nidra. Maharishi Patanjali describes Sleep as a distinct mental state – one which is different from the meditative state he discusses later in the text. It can be unexpected for many to consider Sleep as a mental state that may be controlled and subdued.

When the mind is in the Sleep state, all the external inputs are switched off. We do not hear or see anything, neither the sense of touch is processed. Even the spatial awareness is not present. The body is partially paralysed so that we may not hurt ourselves in sleep. We lose all sense of body, the surrounding and reality (as we know it) itself. The mind turns inwards and if it is a good night's sleep, there is absolutely no perception of passing of time the next morning. In this state there is no content or idea to support the mind.

Sleep is a very powerful state and one that is necessary for survival. There is a reason this habit is exhibited by all living creatures. Good sleep is necessary for repair of wear and tear of the body and brain. There are some functions that can take place only in deep sleep – for example the removal of the waste that the brain produces in the waking state, making neural connections that help in creativity and memory, and dreaming which is physiologically and psychologically vital.

One must not misinterpret this sutra that sleep is unnecessary. In Bhagavad Gita, Shri Krishna mentions moderate sleep as one of the parameters of achieving success on the path of Yoga. Sleep should be regulated. Sleep which is at a proper time, for an appropriate number of hours brings clarity and energy in the waking state, and is immensely desirable. Undesirable is the sleep that makes us feel dull all day long, and robs us of the keenness of the mind.

1.11

DON'T YOU REMEMBER?

अनुभूतविषयासम्प्रमोषः स्मृतिः ॥
anubhūtaviṣayāsampramoṣaḥ smṛtiḥ ॥
(Anubhut-vishaya Asampramosha Smriti)

That which is solely from the past and has not faded; is Memory.

"Memory is like a treadmill. It gives you a lot of exercise, but never takes you anywhere." -Sadhguru

Memory, the fifth vritti of the mind, is the most recognizable vrittis of all. As our life goes on and we continue to experience events and emotions, the brain stores these events. Memory is what allows us to experience Time, for it provides a frame of reference to measure change.

Every event that we experience has an emotional context. A heartbreak is painful, a wedding brings joy, and a loss of loved one causes grief. Emotions not only affect our psyche, but also our physiology. If these emotions are not dealt with in a healthy way, and are not allowed to resolve, they stay stored in the tissues of the body. It is a comment phenomenon for body pains, and irregularities to surface when a memory is accessed. When our mind accesses the memory and remembers the event, the emotions associated with the event surface along with the details of the event. The mind is not able to distinguish between a memory and reality – it reacts the same way as if it was going through the event in the present moment.

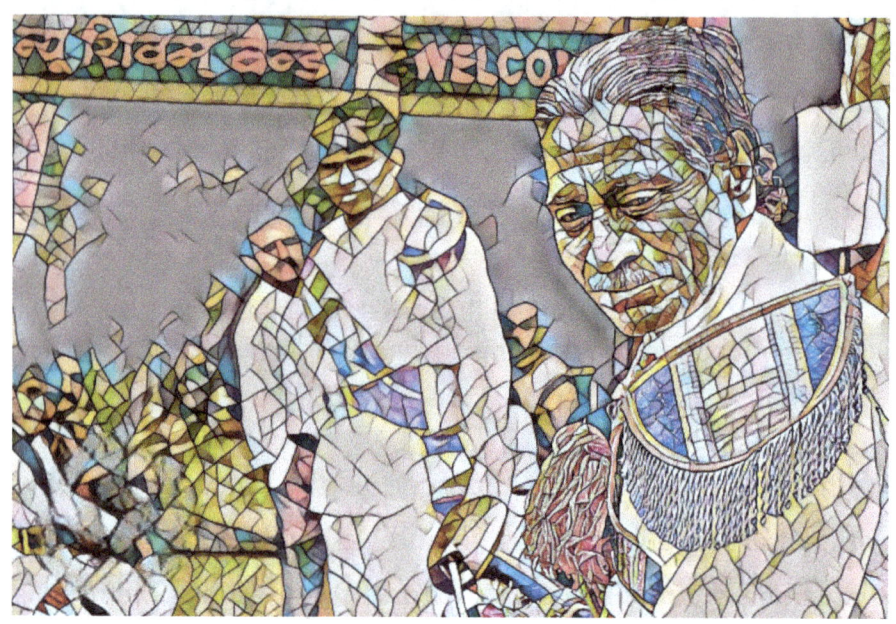

In fact, more the intensity of our emotions at the time of the event, it is more likely the memory is really solid in our body and brain. Psychologists and sleep scientists have found that dreaming about a traumatic event helps in deleting the emotional context of an undesirable event and hence helps in moving on from that event. Now dreaming is possible only in deep states of sleep, and that requires relaxation of some kind. Therefore, in essence, a relaxed mind, is more likely to heal and move on. The past, while it serves to make better decision in the future, must be at beck and call, and not something that should invade the mind anytime it wants. Memory should be a powerful tool, an instrument to navigate the world – it should not become a burden that prevents movement. Unfortunately, this happens to all of us. There are so many memories that we wish we did not have, and there are so many events we wish we could relive – both futile desires.

The past does not exist. There are also many instances in daily life when the past shadows the present. If you had once a bad experience with a roller coaster ride, it is very likely you get a bad taste in your mouth when you see them today. Most of the people will not get along with people they started with on a wrong foot. A person, who wins a few games at a gambling, has higher chances of becoming an addict than him who does not win the games initially. The memory overpowers the intellect, and affects the decision making and experiences of the present. Therefore, this vritti needs to be controlled if one wishes for clarity in perception and awareness.

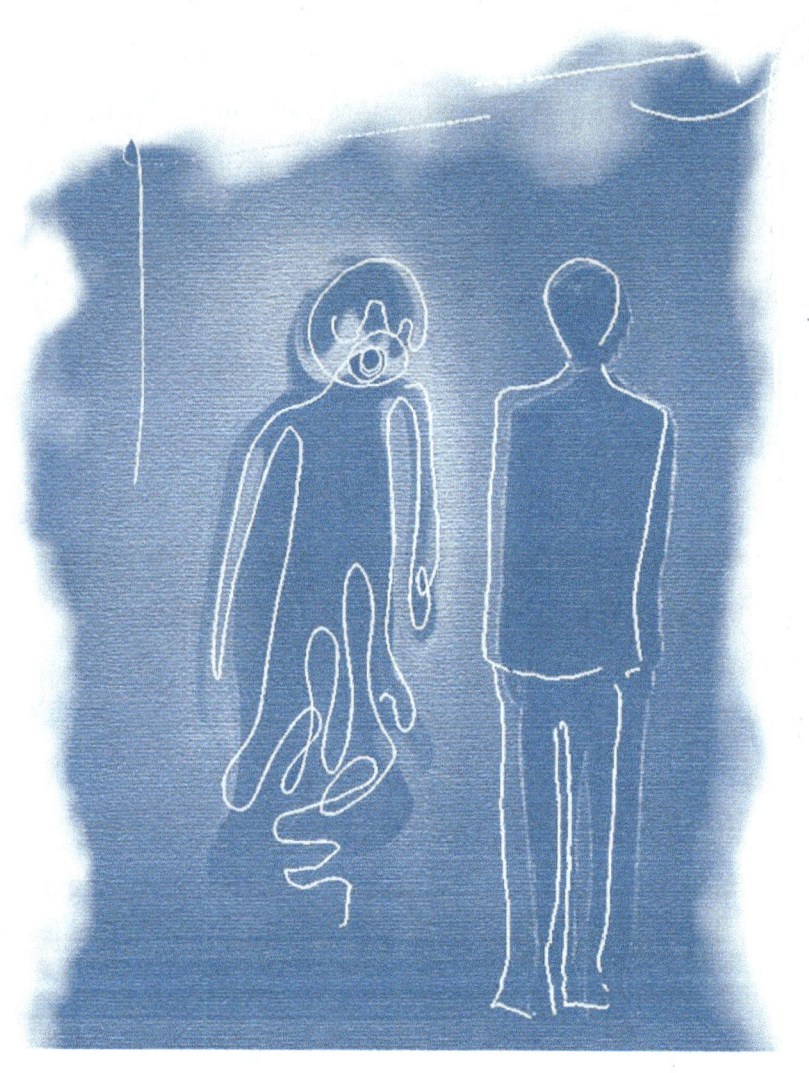

1.12

THE TWIN TOWERS

अभ्यासवैराग्याभ्यां तन्निरोधः ॥
abhyāsavairāgyābhyāṁ tannirodhaḥ ॥
(Abhyasa Vairagya-bhyam Tat Nirodha)

By the application of Abhyasa (Practice) and Vairagya (Dispassion); are those tempered.

"I directed our focus less to the prize of victory than to the process of improving…I knew if I did that, winning would take care of itself."
-Bill Walsh

The mind is not easy to tame. What an understatement! How many times have we given to habits and temptations? How many new year resolutions forgotten? How many promises to ourselves to become better broken? It is not that we do not want to become better, it is just that we are unable. We, as a generation, consume more self-help information than any other. It has not made much of a difference, except for robbing us of our autonomy of intellect and decision-making. We all are looking for someone to tell us how to live. We all are ready to live second-hand lives. Fortunately, and unfortunately, it does not work this way. Listening to someone will never make a difference. Motivation will never last. Focusing only on the goal will seldom lead anyone to achieve the goal. Consistent effort, without attachment to the goal is what yields results. There is no other secret, or key. Abyasa encompasses discipline, consistency, and enjoying the process. When Abhyasa is proper, dispassion flowers on its own.

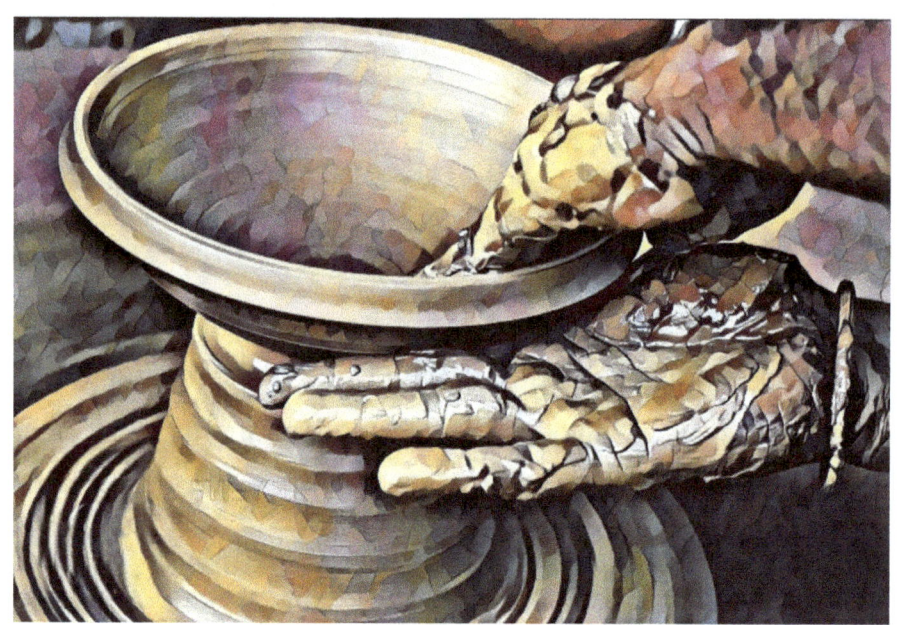

1.13

THE PRACTICE OF PRACTICE

तत्र स्थितौ यत्नोऽभ्यासः ॥
tatra sthitau yatno'bhyāsaḥ ॥
(Tatra stitha yatna Abhyasa)

Being constant and dedicated in one's efforts is Abhyasa.

"How do you expect great things to happen if you are not willing to give your everything to what you wish to do in life." – SADHGURU

Have you ever dissolved into some activity? It may be something at work, studying, playing an instrument, playing a sport, or reading a book? If I ask you to describe your environment at that time, you will draw a blank. You weren't even aware of your body, your consciousness, or time. In those hours, there were no modulations in the mind. The mind had coalesced and become one pointed. Abhyasa does not simply means Practice – it means excellency in practice. Excellence demands regular effort, practice without excuses. The practice must become as much a part of ourselves as breathing, eating, or sleeping. Then Abhyasa bears fruit. Then greatness is not achieved, it simply comes.

We have been told again and again multiple times since our childhood that the mind is a mischievous fellow – it cannot be brought under control. We say things like "Oh, I just could not control the urge" or "I went wandering with my thoughts" or "My mind simply refuses to do it." We have given up the responsibility of the mind. We have such a powerful tool that is not bound by the constraints of space and time and we have given up on it. How can we give up on our gift? We have all accepted that the state of the mind is its own doing and not ours. Where is the mind? Isn't the mind a part of us? Just like we take responsibility for the health of our body, we need to accept responsibility for the health of our mind too. Let us become aware of the thoughts that bother us and do not need any attention. Let us make it a practice of letting them go. There are habits that do need our time, that do not bring any joy. Let us practice giving them up. It sounds difficult – it is difficult, but it is so because we did not know it can be done and hence have maybe never tried it. Let us dissolve into the practice, again and again, until it becomes our very nature.

P.S - I highly recommend attending the Samatvam course conducted by Krishan Verma. I have found tremendous will power and clarity of the way of the mind by attending this course. The simple yet profound knowledge is the need of the hour. You can explore his website below and subscribe to receive notifications for the upcoming courses.

Shudham-Waves of Pure Yoga
https://shudham.org/upcoming-programs/

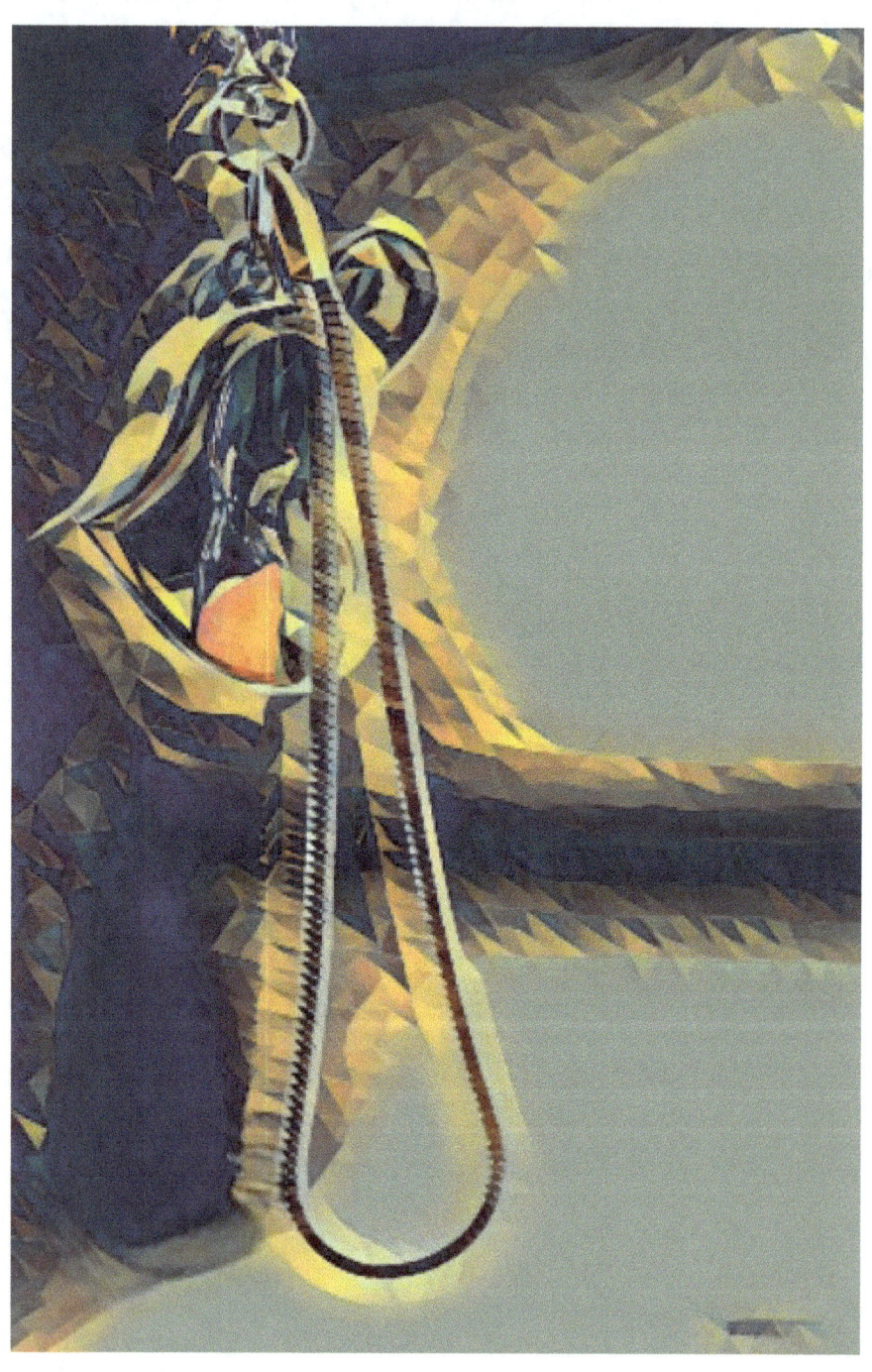

1.14

THE NATURE OF PRACTICE

स तु दीर्घकालनैरन्तर्यसत्कारासेवितो दृढभूमिः ॥
sa tu dīrghakālanairantaryasatkārāsevito dṛḍhabhūmiḥ ॥
(Sa tu Dirgha-kala Nairantarya, Satkara-asevita, Dridhabhumi)

When a practice is Done for a long time incessantly, and with honor; it establishes firm foundation for a powerful life.

"We are what we repeatedly do. Excellence, then, is not an act, but a habit."
-Will Durant

Uninterrupted practice requires extraordinary discipline. It needs sacrifices. It needs setting the priorities straight. It needs will power to power through the bad days and the days "we don't feel like it." An athlete practices for years at a stretch to win that one medal, a musician practices every day to become one with the music and to create something integral that resonates with the soul and is new. Painters paint for years, every day, hoping for one masterpiece to be created from their brush. And when the great event happens, they will tell you that they did not do it and that it just happened. For it to just happen, one needs to do for a very long time, uninterrupted.

How can one keep on practicing if the results are not assured? It may sound cliché here, but it is the process that is important – practicing for years and not giving up makes a champion, not winning a medal. Letting the art consume you makes you a good artist, not becoming famous. To undertake such a process, one needs respect for the practice. You can give your 100% if you respect the practice – then you will not be distracted and also it will be a priority. You need to honor the practice because it reflects honoring your own time, your own Self.

Sachin Tendulkar, the great cricketer, and endearingly referred to as 'The Master Blaster' and the 'God of Cricket', the latter popular in India, has in many interviews talked about the immense respect for his game. He worshipped the game and made sure that all his actions reflected the greatness of the game and in turn he became a figure of worship for the millions of fans of cricket around the world and a great advocate of the game. If you think about it, he just hits a ball with a bat, and he does it better than others. It is the effort, time and discipline that went into becoming better over two decades that has won him the respect and adulation from around the globe.

Valentino Rossi, considered by many the greatest Moto GP racer of all time and winner of 8 World Championships, sits with his motorcycle and "talks" to it before every race. If you see some of the races he has won, you will see he instantly caresses the bike, thanking it for its effort. The motorcycle has in return brought him unparalleled love and affection – from all over the world, even though many great racers have dominated the game across generations.

I have observed many Indian Musical Maestros to actually bow down to the instrument they play before picking it up every day. Similarly, we are to practice the art of reigning in the mind. We have let the mind take control for our entire lives, and it is unrealistic to hope that we can control it overnight. This practice will also take time. One needs to respect the mind and its nature. If the practice is intermittent, the connection is broken. It is like body-building – you cannot go the gym 1 day a week and then expect your muscles to grow. The muscles lose the strength that you build in that one day. Similarly, the mind needs the practice every day, repeatedly, as often as possible without a gap.

In due course of time does one reap the fruit of such a practice. Equanimity and strength become nature. The roots of Yoga take hold in the personality and the true nature comes forth shining.

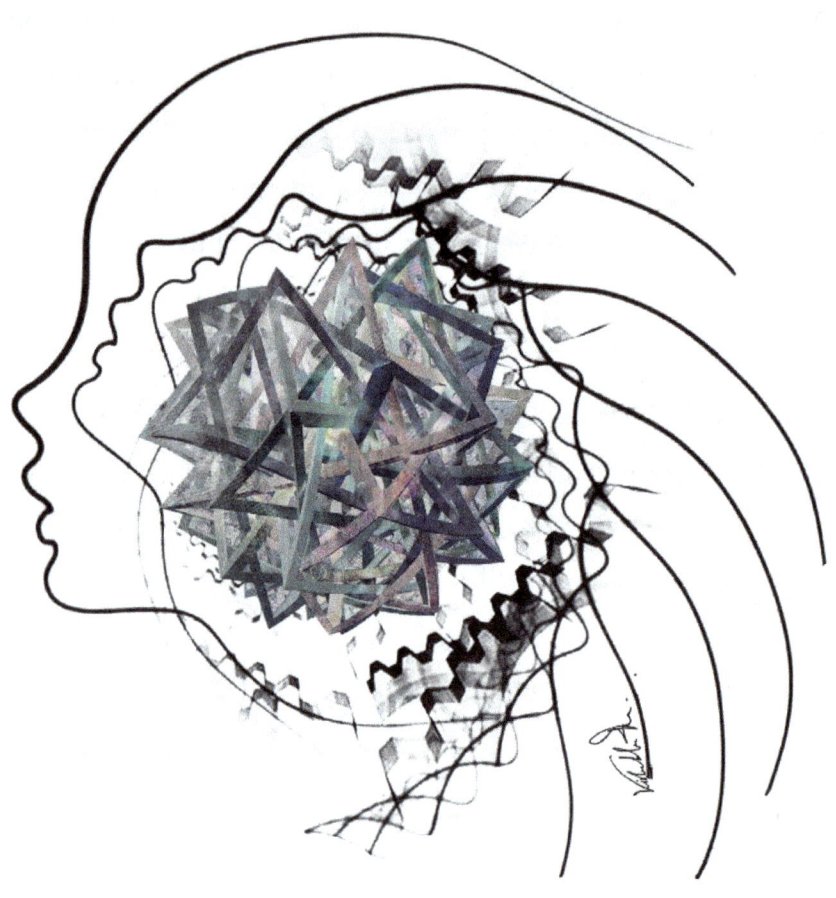

1.15

THE PARADOX OF DETACHMENT

दृष्टानुश्रविकविषयवितृष्णस्य वशीकारसंज्ञा वैराग्यम् ॥
dṛṣṭānuśravikaviṣayavitṛṣṇasya vaśīkārasaṁjñā vairāgyam ॥
(Drishta Anushravika Vishaya vitrshnasya vashikara, sangya Vairagya)

Being able to keep the feverishness in check for the sensual pleasures experienced and heard (including memory and intuition); is Vairagya.

"Vairgaya is not a habit. It is an awareness."
- Sri Sri Ravi Shankar

It is basic human nature to seek joy that lasts because untainted joy is our very self. We run towards some thing or the another and run away from other things. We are troubled by that which give us pleasure and also which give us misery for both these objects shake us from our center. The world trains us to label things as desirable and undesirable, superior and inferior, good and bad, happy and sad, and in turn we keep on vacillating between pleasure and misery without finding anything that lasts.

We do not realize that things are not the answer for the void that consumes each one us. People either get stuck on some sensory experience they had had in their lifetime and are unable to be peaceful because they wish to experience that same joy again and again, or some believe that there is something that someone else has experienced and told them about which is the only thing that will bring them joy and hence they stay miserable as they consider themselves unlucky. At the other end of the spectrum, the mind sticks to something it does not like and fails to find peace. Like and dislike come from a limited perspective. We all have preferences but letting that preferences control us obscure the reality of the event. These likes and dislikes do not allow the mind to focus and settle and such a life is spent in conflict.

Vairagya is a difficult word to understand. It has been interpreted in so many ways by different schools and different teachers that many people bolt at the mention of this word. A person who dons orange clothes and gives up the normal lifestyle and lives the life of a monk is called a Vairagi (one who has attained Vairagya) by many. Many believe that practicing Vairagya means giving up family, wealth and a comfortable life and spending time begging or chanting "Aum" in the caves of the Himalayas. Others believe that becoming emotionless is Vairagya. A person who does not care for his parents, his friends, and other people around him and is always stoic and serious is called Vairagi by many because Vairagya is translated as detachment. What a foolish thought. What a sad life.

Vairagya is a state of mind – one of dispassion, one of stability, one of enthusiasm, one of joy that is not based on any external factor. There is no love greater than that of a Vairagi for he loves without a reason, because it is his very nature. There is no person more efficient and enthusiastic in action because the action does not need to accomplish anything to be joyful – his inner joy makes the action joyful. He will fulfil every duty towards everyone with utmost devotion because such a person shall take responsibility for everything and everyone around him. He will be the greatest asset of a civilization. Pleasure and pain, happiness and sadness, success and failure fail to impact him because he is aware of the temporary nature of duality. Vairagya dawns itself when there is discipline, and consistency. Vairagya is unparalleled bliss.

1.16

TRANSCENDING TRINITY

तत्परं पुरुषख्यातेर्गुणवैतृष्ण्यम् ॥
tatparaṁ puruṣakhyāterguṇavaitṛṣṇyam ॥
(Tatparam Purusha, khyate Guna, Vaitrshnyam)

Highest Vairagya is achieved when one gets in touch with the Purusha (the highest consciousness); which happens when the Trigunas lose their influence.

"There is no joy that Vairagya cannot beget you."
-Adi Shankaracharya

A person who has achieved Vairagya can keep his focus, and does not deviate from his path. But even in this state, the trigunas influence each emotion, thought and action.

The Samkhya philosophy (one of the six Indian philosophies) gives the concept of Prakriti – the manifest, that interacts with Purusha - the supreme consciousness. Prakriti is made of 3 aspects – Inertness/Rest (Tamas), Dynamism/Action (Rajas), and Stability/Focus (Sattva) which are called the Trigunas. Each and every aspect of the Nature (prakriti) is affected by the Trigunas.

The human mind is also driven by these three qualities. It is no mere co-incidence we refer to a person's temperament as their "nature." Each individual has a certain attitude towards life they are born with – some are lazy, some are restless, and some are stable in their directions and are balanced. People are a combination of these qualities and a particular quality dominates at different times of the day, month, and year. Food and environment also play a major role in which quality dominates in an individual.

A person high in Sattva would have clarity in his mind, and would be emotionally healthy and stable, and energetic. A person high in Rajas would be dynamic, unable to rest, his mind shooting in multiple directions at a time causing confusion. Tamas brings laziness and too much of it causes dullness. Do not think that we should do with a quality we do not desire.

Each quality is necessary for balance. Without Tamas, one would not be able to sleep, too much of Rajas causes conflict and too little of it causes inaction. Too much of Sattva is beneficial only when one is doing some higher practice – otherwise it can affect the mind in undesirable ways if not handled properly. If one understands this, one starts observing what is causing distress, moodiness, and passion. We can get out of blaming ourselves and others.

There are rare people who can transcend even the basic impulses of the human life. With Abhyasa, Vairagya, and grace of the Guru, such people realize the Self. Realizing and experiencing oneself as the Purusha is the higher Vairagya. Here the "I" vanishes and then only each and every particle is recognized as a part of the Self. In the higher form of Vairagya, there are no desires left in the individual. Hunger, thirst, fear, anger, greed, and lust are eradicated and no latent impressions guide the decisions.

The three gunas – Sattva, Rajas, and Tamas do not have any influence on the individual. They dissolve as they have fulfilled their purpose of becoming one with the Purusha. The individual truly achieves freedom in every aspect in this world and beyond.

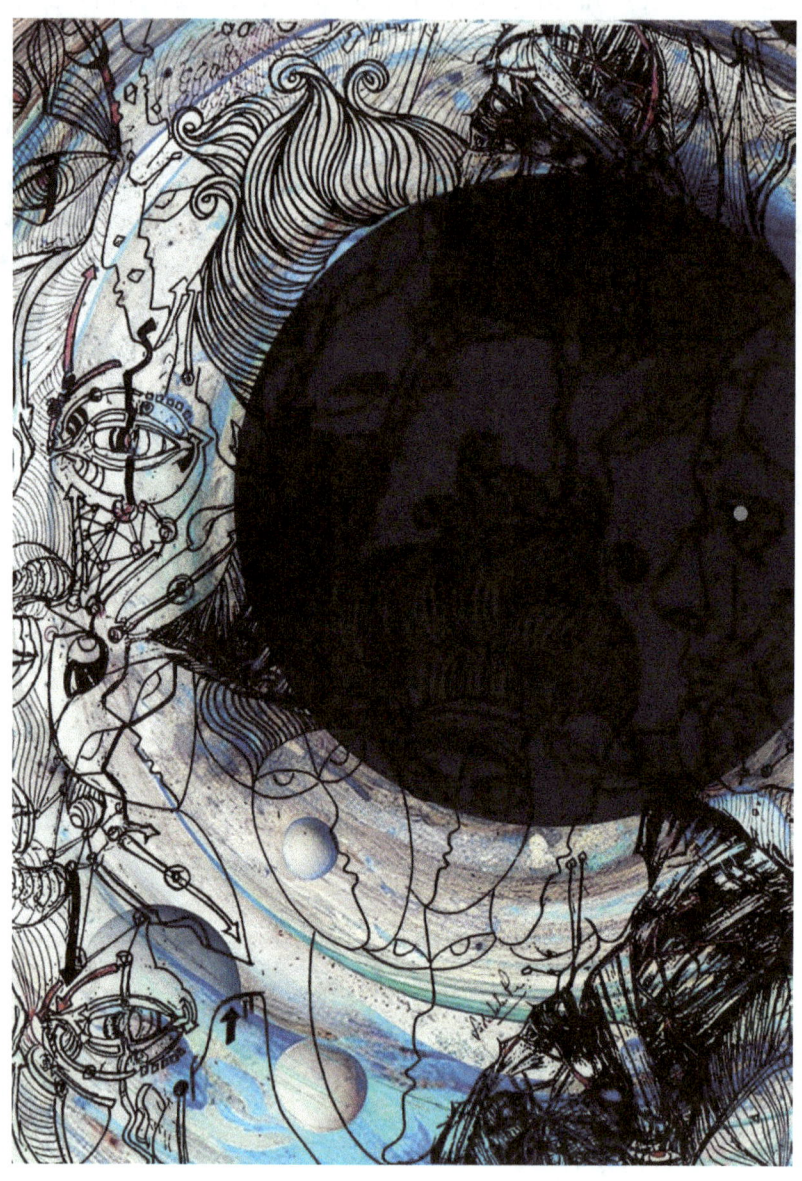

1.17

HALF-AWAKE

वितर्कविचारानन्दास्मितारूपानुगमात् सम्प्रज्ञातः ॥
vitarkavicārānandāsmitārūpānugamāt samprajñātaḥ ॥
(Vitarka Vichaara Ananda Asmita-rupa-anugamaat, Samprajnaata)

Samprajnatah is achieved by Reasoning (vitarka), Reflection (vichara), Bliss (ananda), and Oneness-with-the-object (asmita-rupa-anugamat).

Impressions rise according to the dominant guna (Sattva, Rajas, or Tamas) and affect thoughts, emotions, and consequently decisions and actions. The method to clean the mind is meditation which culminates into Samadhi – a state in which the physical and the pranic plane is transcended, and the mental plane is explored and healed and finally even that is dropped. The state of Samadhi is not akin to sleeping - one is at rest but alert.

According to the science of Yoga, there are five planes of existence that a human being can experience. These are called Panchakosha – The Five Sheaths which envelope the atman – the soul.

Annamaya Kosha – the physical plane. Anna literally means food. The body that is composed of food that we eat and drink is the Annamaya Kosha. Bones, organs, muscles, blood, semen, lymphatic fluid, and plasma all fall under the Annamaya Kosha.

Pranamaya Kosha - the vital energy which courses through the body in psychic channels and transforms in Chakras which are psychic centers. Asana, Pranayama, and other techniques of Prana Vidya (The science of Prana) can help a person to perceive Prana and over time, with regular practice, manipulate it.

Manomaya Kosha– the mental plane. All thoughts and many kinds of impressions lie in this plane. While we all can agree that we have thoughts, very few of us can witness them. It is evident Descartes had never experienced the state of Samadhi when he said "I think, therefore I am." Otherwise, he would have said "I am, therefore I think."

Vijnanamaya Kosha – The intellectual body is the plane of analysis and awareness. Forming judgements, making decisions, weighing pros and cons, and being aware of oneself within and without are the activities of Vijnanamaya Kosha.

Anandamaya Kosha – the plane of bliss and joy. We all have at different times in our life have experienced ecstasy. For that few minutes, one experiences Anandamaya Kosha. Prana, or the vital energy pervades all the sheaths. If it did not, life would not be possible.

For most people, it is not easy to slip into meditation. Most who try are frightened by the onslaught of thoughts the first time. A simple way to slip into meditation is by gathering the mind onto one object. It is called Samprajnatah – the meditation with the support of an object. There are four stages of this samadhi: Reasoning (vitarka), Reflection (vichara), bliss/inspiration (Ananda) and Oneness with object (asmita-rupa). One supports -the mind with an object of choice – it begins with careful examination of the object during which all thoughts except the object disappear, followed by mental contemplation in which the effort is no longer needed to examine the object. In the end the practitioner become one with the object of meditation. Each stage is a progression – layer by - layer the impressions are destroyed and the next layer of impressions take the practitioner into the next stage of Samprajnatah Samadhi.

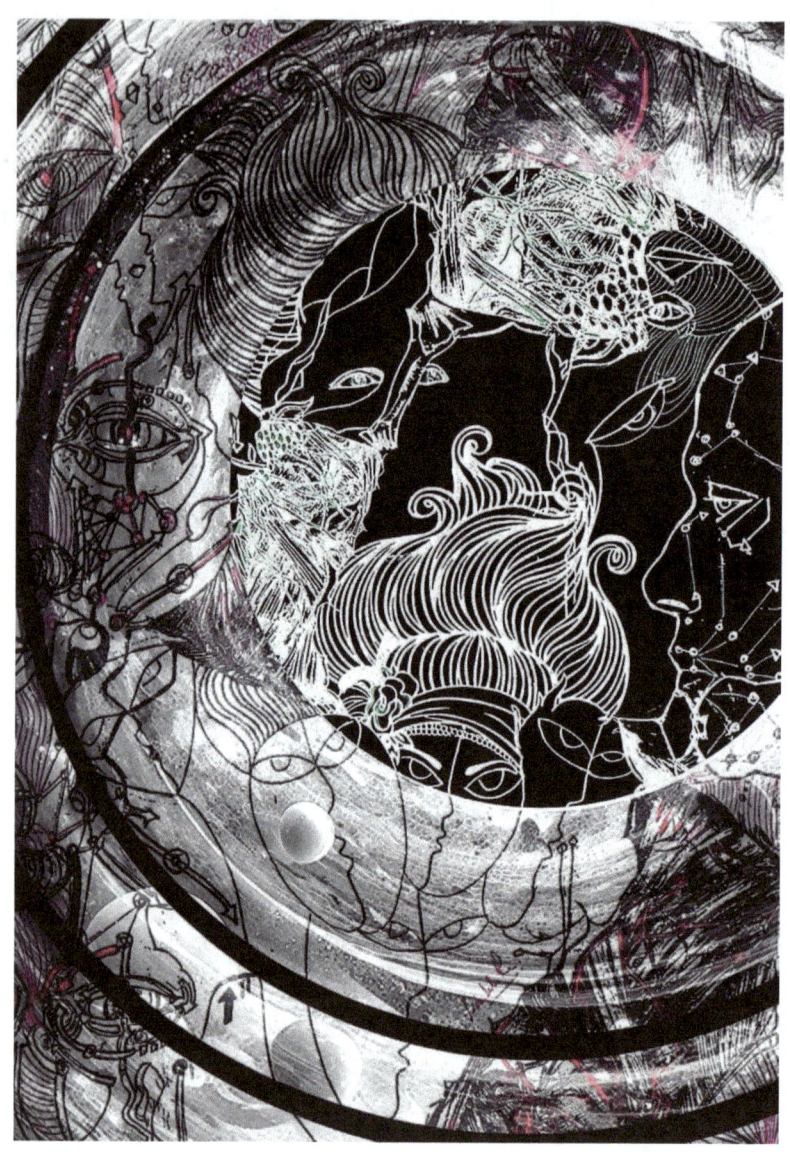

1.18

HALF-ASLEEP

विरामप्रत्ययाभ्यासपूर्वः संस्कारशेषोऽन्यः ॥
virāmapratyayābhyāsapūrvaḥ saṁskāraśeṣo'nyaḥ ॥
(Viraam pratyaya, Abhayaasa-purva, Samskaara-sesa, Anya)

There is an Another type of Samadhi which is achieved due to prior practices. In this state the mind is devoid of content but latent impressions remain.

- asmitā_of_form = Oneness i.e. finally a sense of Oneness prevails

The distinguishing character of Samprajnatah Samadhi is the presence of Pratyaya – content on which the mind is dwelling which can be an object, an idea, a mantra, or even a person (Guru). In all stages of Samprajnatah Samadhi, the object of contemplation exists. As one progresses to different stages of Samprajnatah Samadhi, latent impressions are destroyed.

Samskaras mean impressions that we have collected over our lifetimes – they are the result and further cause of experiences, thoughts, emotions, identities, desires, and all other content of the consciousness. Samskara is called the seed of consciousness by Swami Satyananda Saraswati. Until the Samskaras exist, the consciousness is still not able to experience its infinity. Two broad categories of Samadhi have been given by Maharishi Patanjali: Sabeeja Samadhi and Nirbeeja Samadhi.

Sabeeja literally means "with seed" and Nirbeeja literally means "without seed." Here the seed refers to Samskaras.

Sabeeja Samadhi consists of those states of samadhi in which the Samskaras are still present.

Nirbeeja Samadhi is the highest state of Samadhi – here the very seeds of consciousness have been destroyed and *Kaivalya* (Liberation) has been achieved. Many commentators and authors have reportedly confused this Sutra as describing the Nirbeeja Samadhi. It is not so. This sutra simply talks about the state of Samadhi in which the object is not present but the latent impressions (Samskaras) remain.

The different stages of Samprajnatah Samadhi as given by Maharishi Patanjali in his previous sutra are *Vitarka* (Examination), *Vichara* (Reflection), *Ananda* (Joy), and *Asmita* (Oneness). In between every stage, there is a state in which *Pratyaya* (the object of contemplation) is dropped and mind has no awareness and is tranquil but, the latent impressions are still existing and active.

Asamprajnatah Samadhi may be experienced while progressing from one stage of Samprajnatah Samadhi to another - between Vitarka and Vichara, Vichara and Ananda, and Ananda and Asmita, or may be directly experienced. Therefore, the two distinguishing characteristics to understand Asamprajnatah Samadhi are: dropping of Pratyaya and existence of Samskaras. Asamprajnatah Samadhi may be achieved due to practice of Samprajnatah Samadhi or may result as a fruit of other practices in this lifetime and previous lifetimes. There are many people who experience this state of thoughtlessness without practicing Samprajnatah Samadhi due to other prior practices.

One does not need to analyze the kind of Samadhi that is being achieved because that itself won't allow the practitioner to achieve Samadhi.

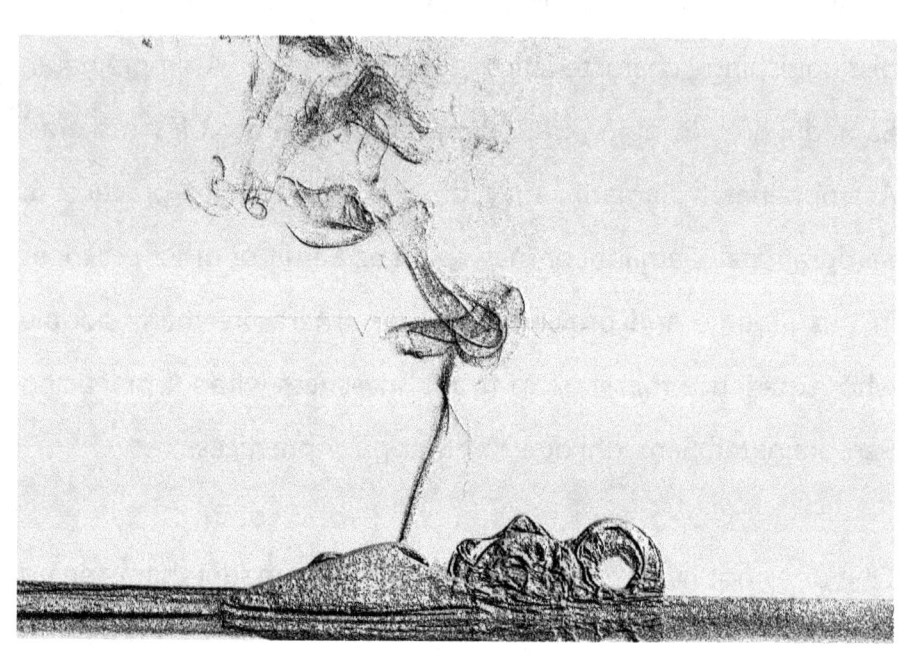

1.19

DISSOLVE

भवप्रत्ययो विदेहप्रकृतिलयानाम् ॥
bhavapratyayo videhaprakṛtilayānām ॥
(Bhava Pratyaya videha, Prakriti laya)

There is a state of meditation achieved only due to past practices (loss of body consciousness); and another in which the mind dissolves in Nature.

"I love not man the less, but Nature more." -Lord Byron

Asamprajnatah Samadhi is achieved by merit – it is possible that the merit was earned in previous lifetimes. In Bhagavad Gita, Shri Krishna tells Arjuna that one who walks on the path of spiritual practice, even if he does not achieve the goal in this lifetime, carries over the merit to the next lifetime and continues from where he left off.

The great saint Ramana Maharishi sat in Samadhi for 6 months in a temple at the young age of 16, and was spoon-fed by the temple priests. Jagadish Vasudev, popularly known as Sadhguru, mentions his experiences with unintentional periods of Samadhi, which on rare occurrence continued for days in his book 'Inner Engineering.' The loss of body consciousness is not limited to food, water or sleep but also includes the sensory urges.

The other type of meditation is one where the person gets absorbed into Nature. You can experiment – just comfortably lie down under a clear blue sky and stare at it. The sleep you will slip into would not be regular sleep. You will experience rest like you have never known.

There is a reason we rush to the mountains or to the sea. We look at the stars and feel like they are calling us home. The sea invites us to its depths - we experience some inkling of the infinity we really are while in Nature. The five elements of the body are purified and harmonize with the same five elements that make up the entire universe. It is as if a fog lifts from the mind. The clarity is sudden. There is a sense of space and vastness. Time seems to stand still.

The world is such a beautiful place that experiencing this state might be one of the easiest states if one takes out some time for experiencing it. The grandiose of the nature reminds us of the bigger picture, uplifts our spirits and satisfies our core. Just watching the sun rise or set every day for 10 minutes can be included in the daily routine – remembering that the same fire that burns in the sun also burns inside us, that the same Space is home to this magnificent star and our magnificent person can be transmogrifying.

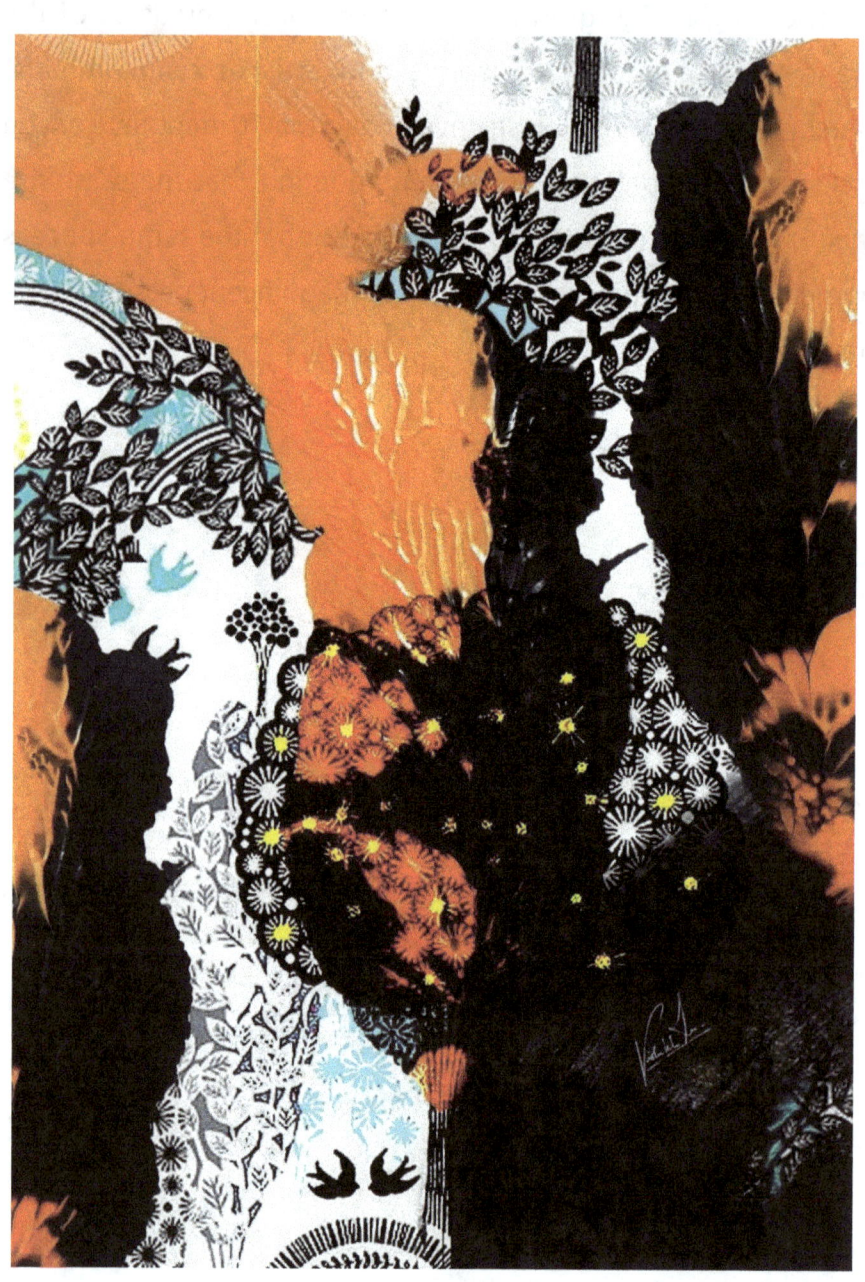

1.20

SOWING SEEDS

श्रद्धावीर्यस्मृतिसमाधिप्रज्ञापूर्वक इतरेषाम् ॥
śraddhāvīryasmṛtisamādhiprajñāpūrvaka itareṣām ॥
(Shraddha Virya Smriti Samadhi Prajna-purvaka Itareshaam)

Others attain Asamprajnatah Samadhi by having Faith, Courage, Memory, and Self-Awareness.

> "Courage is grace under pressure."
> - Ernest Hemmingway

Rare few people can slip into Samadhi without any effort. The rest of the sadhakas have to practice the techniques imparted by their Guru to achieve Meditation.

The first quality needed is Shraddha – Faith. A disciple must have faith in the Master/Guru and the knowledge imparted by Him. Otherwise, the potency of the technique is destroyed by the seed of the doubt.

Doubt can be of three types:
- Doubt on Self
- Doubt on the Master
- Doubt on the Technique

The second quality is Courage. Many people abandon their practices at the first sign of trouble. They believe that if they are on this path, no difficult situation should arise in their lives. Some people get sick and they start complaining – How can we get sick? We do Yoga every day. What is it that I am doing wrong?

The nature of the body is to decay – there are going to be sick days, but if you are doing your Sadhana, you will recover quickly, and there won't be any long-term effect of the sickness. Similarly, the nature of the mind is to wander: it will be exhausted some days without reason but these days will be fewer for those established in a regular practice. Sadhana is not a means to escape. All types of situations are going to come.

Sadhana builds endurance and patience, and helps overcome misery and grief before it makes any lasting impression. After some degree of success is achieved, a Sadhak may even be able to witness his emotions like an observer. But if courage is not present, and one starts complaining after stubbing a toe, then it is not extremely difficult to gain the fruit of the Sadhana and experience stillness of Samadhi.

The third quality is Memory. If Samadhi is experienced once, it is possible to use the memory of that experience to slip into Samadhi again. It is one of the easiest ways of going into meditation.

The last quality is putting effort in gaining some amount of self-awareness. The senses are always turned outwards. Simply allowing ourselves to sit and do nothing for a few minutes, to accept and reflect would do wonders.

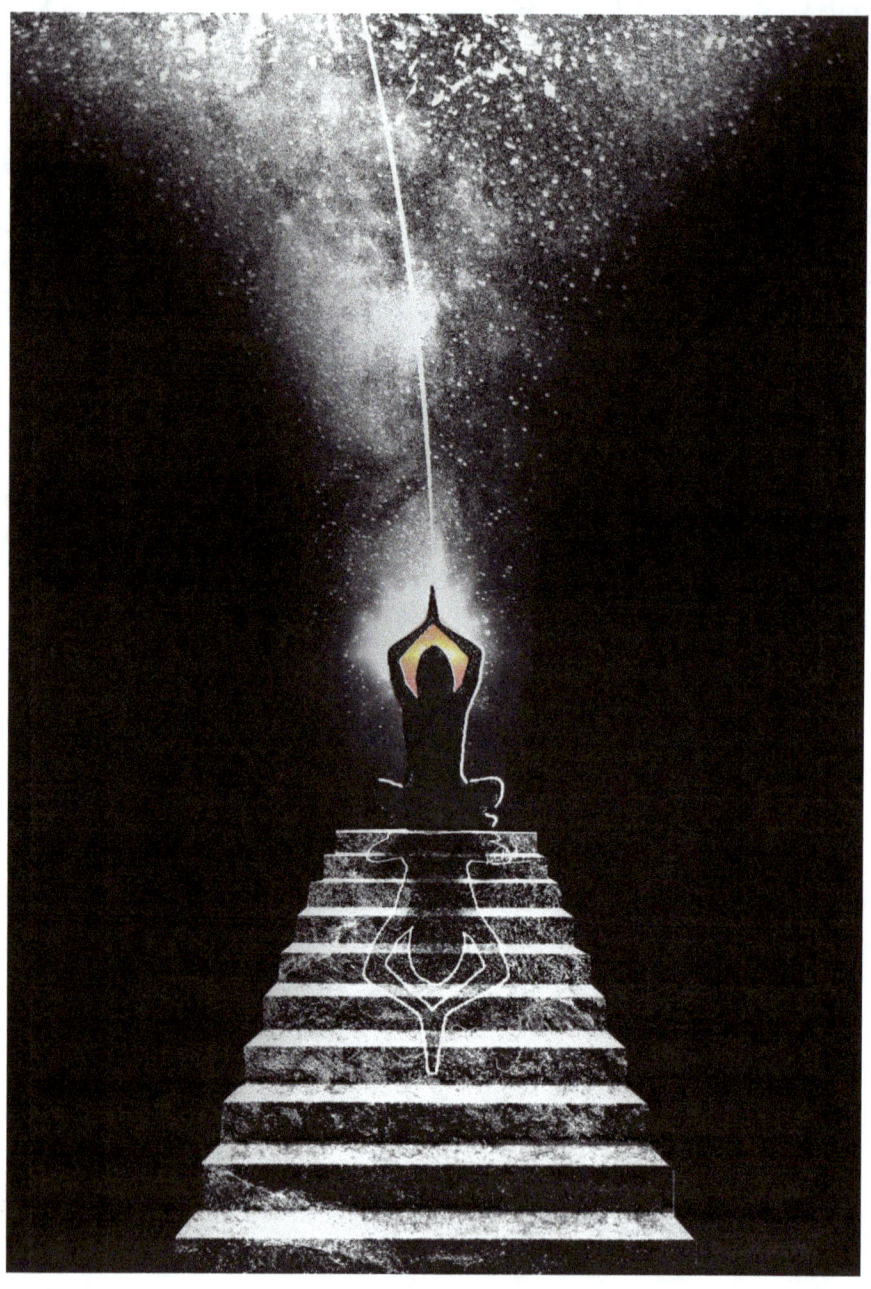

1.21

A CALL TO THE UNIVERSE

तीव्रसंवेगानामासन्नः ॥
tīvrasaṁvegānāmāsannaḥ ॥
(Tivra Samvegana Aasanna)

An intense desire for Liberation; shortens the path to Liberation.

I remember listening to a story when I was a little boy. A young ambitious boy went to a saint and asked him the secret to success. The saint was in Silence and did not answer. This continued for many days. Then one day, the boy decided to follow the saint in the morning and ask him the question when there were no disciples around.

He followed the saint to the river, and as the saint was coming out after bathing, he repeated his question. The saint beckoned the boy towards him. The boy happily entered the river, thrilled with anticipation of the answer. As soon as the boy reached the saint, he grabbed him by his neck and pushed his head under the water. The boy thrashed; his lungs burned. When he finally thought he would black out, the saint pulled him up and said

"The day you want to be successful as badly as you wanted to breathe, you will be successful."

Thoughts are powerful. More focused the thought, more powerful it becomes, and greater is the chance of manifestation. In Pujas and Yajnas, we take Sankalpa – we meditate on our desire, make it strong and surrender into the sacrificial fire. Then no more time is spent thinking about the fulfilment of the desire, but only on efforts. There is a component of Karma Yoga here – the fruit is surrendered to the universe, and when that is done, action becomes more efficient and effective.

If we have an intense desire to achieve success in anything in our life, then we must make it our top-most priority. We must give it your best portion of energy and time. That intense desire makes the success manifest faster. If a Sadhaka has an intense desire to achieve Yoga, he shall achieve it earlier than others. Eagerness, combined with Faith is necessary, perhaps even more necessary than the correct application of the technique for Grace follows Faith and Eagerness. But it must be taken care that the Eagerness does not transform into feverishness.

There is a thin line and it must not be crossed – Vairagya must be developed simultaneously to keep us grounded in the present.

1.22

MORE SUGAR MORE SWEETNESS

मृदुमध्याधिमात्रत्वात् ततोऽपि विशेषः ॥
mṛdumadhyādhimātratvāt tato'pi viśeṣaḥ ॥
(Mridu Madhya Adhimaatratvaat tatopi vishesha)

Urge to achieve Liberation can be of Weak, Medium, or High intensity.

"Most people overestimate what they can achieve in a year, and underestimate what they can achieve in ten years." - Amara's Law

There can be 3 types of people eager for achieving success on this path:

- With weak intensity desire – such people do not prioritize Sadhana. It is something that is done if free time can be found.
- With mild intensity desire – such people may start with a high intensity but are unable to keep up the motivation and it fizzles out. They do not give the utmost priority to their Sadhana. The time and efforts given is average.

- With high intensity desire – they give the highest priority to their Sadhana and achieve success earliest.

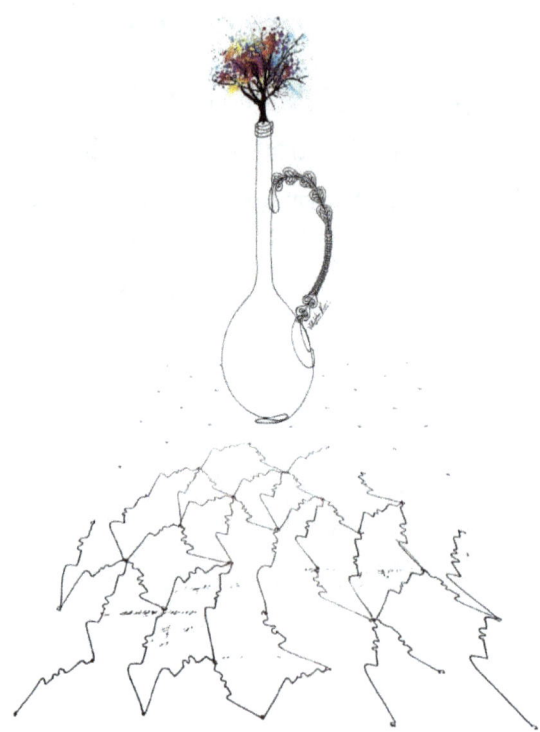

This quality is not limited to only Yoga Sadhana but with any goal in life. If one reads about the extraordinarily successful people, we find they went beyond the normal structure of daily routine. They worked long hours, and did not focus on anything else at all. They follow this routine for a long, long time, but the success they achieve is nothing less than supernatural. Elon Musk, Cristiano Ronaldo, Virat Kohli and Late Dr. APJ Abdul Kalam (former President of India) are fine examples. I had a teacher in my college who had worked under Dr. Kalam in the DRDO Lab and he used to tell stories about Dr. Kalam. He said Dr. Kalam had no sense of day or night, and seemingly operated without food and sleep. The lab he used to enter, that staff knew they may not get to go home that night. He never married. He took the Indian Space Program and Missile Programs to unprecedented heights.

The intensity of the desire manifests into efforts. In the earlier Sutras, Maharishi Patanjali mentions the importance of revering the practice. If one has a strong intensity of desire, reverence automatically comes. One is grateful for the knowledge bestowed by the Guru and make it a priority to practice Sadhana. That which you honor brings you honor in return. Hence, the sadhana fructifies early. Those with average motivation just need a follow up of the knowledge after some time again and again. They will take some more time to achieve success. Those who do not prioritize it at all may or may not achieve any success unless the Guru bestows His Grace. Without any intention to achieve success, one cannot work towards any goal for a long time and hence it cannot be successful unless Luck strikes. It must be understood here that high intensity of desire does not mean a higher Sadhana. A simple practice that a Guru has imparted to the disciple, if done with reverence, honor and faith will take the participant close to achieving Samadhi. Neither does the intensity translate to impatience, for impatience breeds frustration which leads to imbalance in the mind. All other responsibilities must be fulfilled too, but the priority must be set according to situation and age.

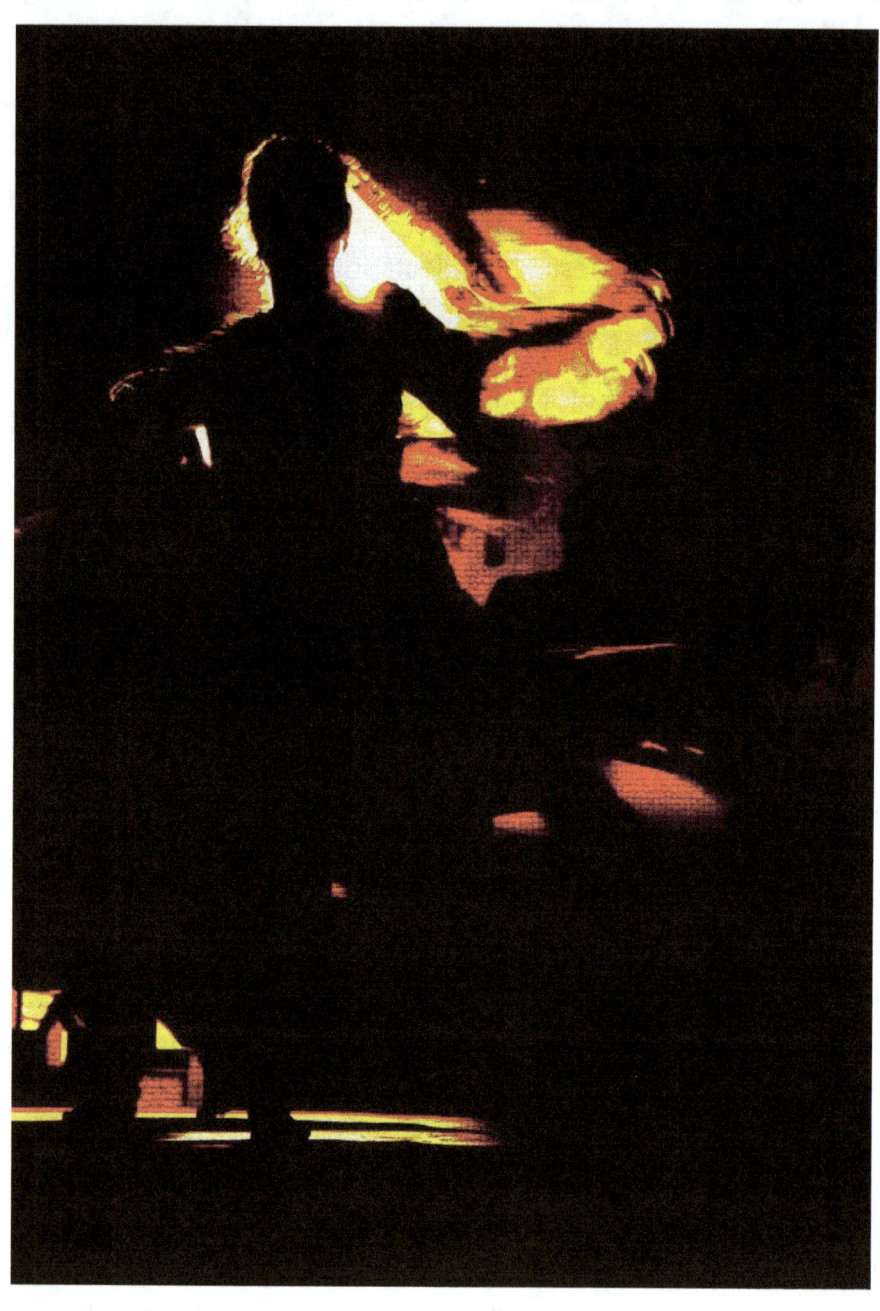

1.23

TRUMP CARD

ईश्वरप्राणिधानाद्वा ॥
īśvarapraṇidhānādvā ॥
(Ishvara pranidhanad vaa)

**Or by total surrender to the Lord
(one can attain success on this path).**

"The ultimate act of power is surrender."
- Krishna Das

Some people achieve the goal of Sadhana at birth or early in life due to Sadhana of the past lifetimes. Some achieve it by the Grace of the Guru – a glance of the Master is enough to take the devotee to the highest plane if the Guru wishes. Others must put in effort for a long time with sincerity and honor.

Some people's minds are not constituted for effort, or their circumstances do not allow them to focus on their spiritual practices. They must not feel hapless, for even these people must have faith to achieve success on the path of Yoga. Such people must surrender themselves totally to God in all respects.

If you believe in Jesus, surrender to Jesus. If you believe in Lord Buddha, surrender to him. Yoga has nothing to do with religion.

For those who believe in a higher intelligence, have faith in that intelligence. Every religion aims to take the person to a higher state of awareness and a more joyful living. The highest entity you believe in is your God. Surrender to that entity. Be completely devoted to them in both thought and action. The last sutra was in context with Karma Yoga. This sutra combines Karma Yoga and Bhakti Yoga. It asks the aspirant to perform all actions and fulfil all responsibilities and dedicate all these actions to God. This is to make sure the aspirant does not drop everything and just sit in the temple. All responsibilities are to be fulfilled. Simultaneously, believing whatever is happening is the will of God, and performing actions without any expectations surely takes the aspirant into Samadhi.

In Bhagavad Gita, Lord Krishna tells Arjuna:
सर्वधर्मान्परित्यज्य मामेकं शरणं व्रज । अहं त्वां सर्वपापेभ्यो मोक्षयिष्यामि मा शुचः ॥
Abandon all Dharmas and surrender to me alone.
I shall liberate you from all sins; do not fear. (Chapter 18, verse 66)

Shri Krishna gives Arjuna a sure shot way. He asks him to forget all that he has learned from the scriptures, forget the code of life he believes is the right way to earn merit for it can be confusing and requires effort. All Arjuna needs to do is to devote himself wholly to Him, and he shall be liberated.

They say Bhakti Yoga is the sweetest path to Liberation. The intoxication of experiencing God leaves no space for any practice and knowledge and neither it is needed. Famous examples are Mirabai, Tulsidas, Kabirdas, Surdas, etc. My yoga teacher Yogacharaya Krishan Vermaji tells to experience oneness with God. All other yoga practices are just attempting to provide this experience only. Remembering God is the most powerful practice.

Ishwar Pranidhana is not only for those with a weak resolve or unfavorable circumstances, it is for every practitioner because Surrendering to God is needed to progress on the journey.

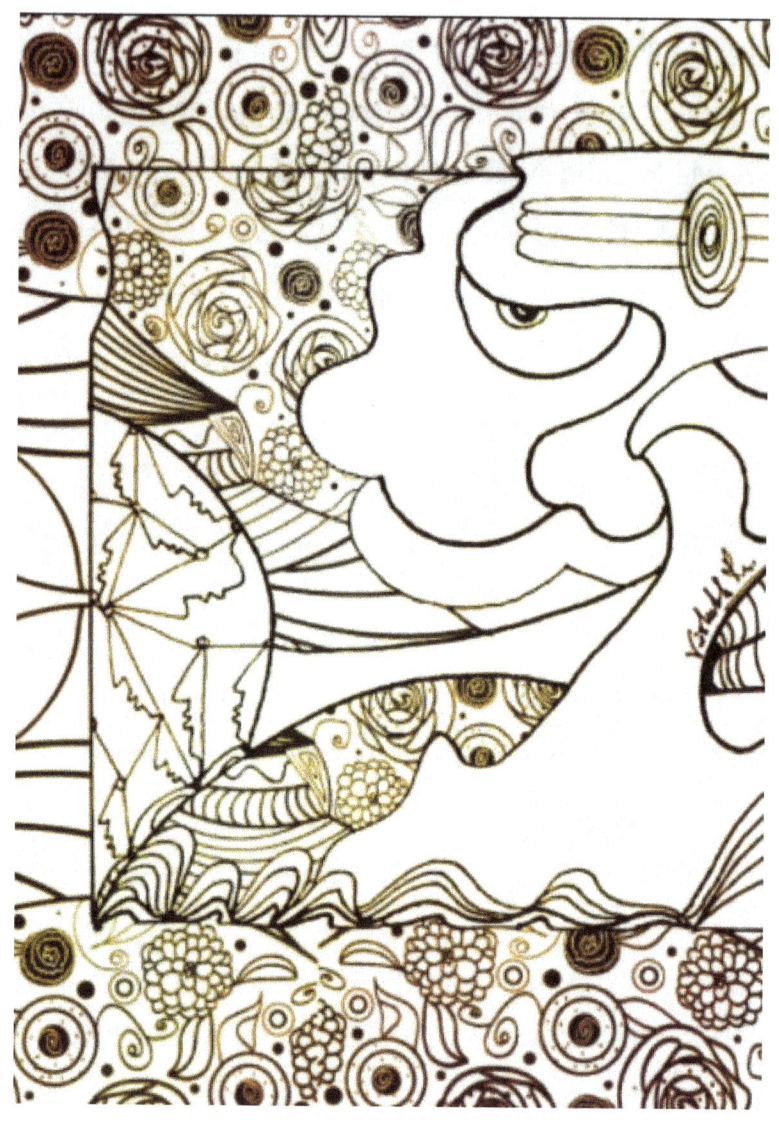

1.24

THE GOD PARTICLE

क्लेशकर्मविपाकाशयैरपरामृष्टः पुरुषविशेष ईश्वरः ॥
kleśakarmavipākāśayairaparāmṛṣṭaḥ puruṣaviśeṣa īśvaraḥ ॥
(Klesha Karma Vipaak-ashayeh, Aparamrishta, Purusha-vishesha Ishvara)

God is One who is untouched by suffering, karma, doership, its impressions and fruits, and holds no expectations.

"God is always the first person, the I, ever standing before you." - Bhagvan Ramana Maharishi

When one mentions God, everyone has a different reaction to it. For some God is a Father sitting in heaven who is categorizing each action and thought as good or evil, and passes judgement after Death. For someone else, God is what we call Soul. For an atheist, this anthropomorphic entity is a farce, created to bully people into doing things which might be against their nature. The words of Cristopher Hitchens "Religion is the root of all Evil" ring true for a lot of people, especially millennials. His argument that there is no good human quality that would not exist without religion is undebatable. But this argument is undebatable only if one views religion from the political standpoint – a pseudo group identity with pseudo assets and ego that must be protected at all costs.

God does not belong to any religion – how could it be if we believe God to be infinite. Meanwhile a religion that does not accept other beliefs cannot be infinite. If it is, then there cannot be any conflict with other factions.

The Upanishads say God is simply the supreme consciousness pervading every particle, every atom - the entire cosmos. It calls it Brahman. It is infinite, omniscient and all encompassing. There is no duality – good and bad, right and wrong, night and day – all these relative terms are meaningless for an infinite, timeless entity. Every religion aims to take the human awareness so that this Supreme Consciousness can be experienced, but this goal has been buried under theological totalitarianism.

Maharishi Patanjali, understood the difference in beliefs and opinions of different people regarding the concept of God. He might have known how many people are God-fearing people, believing in a Being just because they are afraid of the uncertainty of Life and Death, and find solace in a Divine Being that will grant them Heaven after Death. In this sutra, he tries to define God.

Maharishi Patanjali's 3 qualities of God:
1. God is untouched by suffering: Suffering arises only when an undesirable state comes, or when a desirable state passes away. Pleasure and Pain, which are temporary are considered permanent, and that which is permanent is lost. God is eternal itself and hence beyond suffering.
2. God is above doership and actions its impressions and expectations of fruit, and fruit of the action: The supreme consciousness is the cosmic will, and yet it is an observer. In the large frame of things, the entity which can observe each perspective and dimension of an event is God. It is omniscient. It observes everything is happening, and does nothing. There is no doership.
3. God does not hold any expectations or any latent impressions: Since there is no impressions of the actions, no expectations arise of any effect of the action. Therefore, God is timeless for it is always in the present moment.

These qualities are mentioned to remind us that we all have the potential to realize God – to recognize that we are the Supreme

Consciousness that is eternal and timeless. We cannot become God, for we already are, we can only realise it and that is the aim of any spiritual practice.

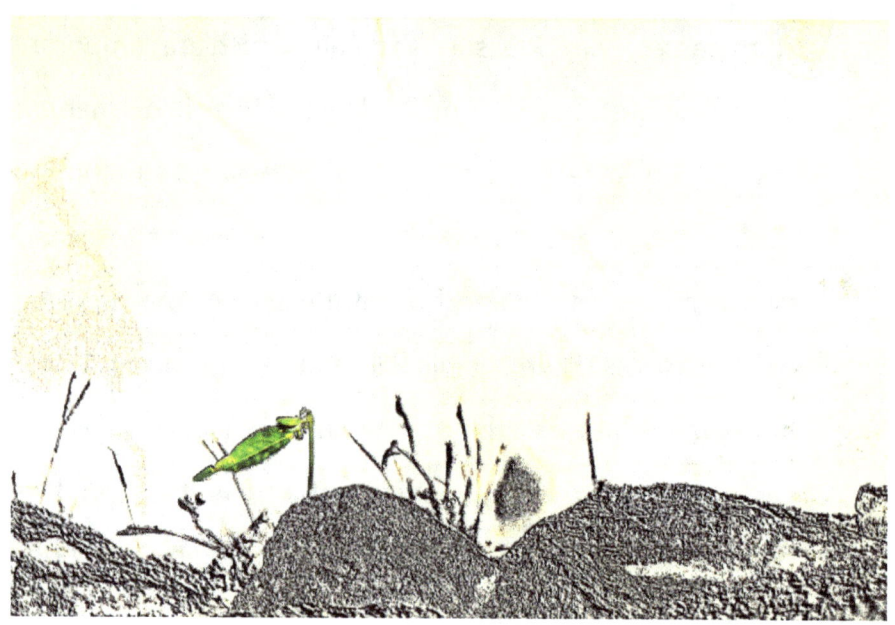

1.25

THE THEORY OF EVERYTHING

तत्र निरतिशयं सर्वज्ञबीजम् ॥
tatra niratiśayaṁ sarvajñabījam ॥
(Tatra niratishaya sarvajna-Bijam)

God is the source from which all Knowledge sprouts.

"What if the solar system was just another atom?"
-A cartoon strip

There is a famous shloka in Yajur Veda "Yat Pinde, Tat Brahmande, Yatha Brahmande Tatha Pinde" – which literally translated means "So is an individual body and so is the cosmos, so is the cosmos and so is an individual body." Here the individual body is not limited to a human body, or the body of an organism, but also refers to the fundamental unit of matter – an atom. The shloka means that if one gains complete knowledge of just one particle of this universe, one will gain the complete knowledge about the entire universe. The microcosm and macrocosm are one fundamentally, no matter how they manifest or act in nature.

The modern theories of the cosmos like String Theory theorize that the entire universe is just one particle at the core of every atom vibrating at different frequencies and manifesting as matter because a consciousness perceives it and causes it to manifest. Modern Science is still trying its best to find the Theory of Everything. The Upanishads gave the same concept including the Theory of Everything with a different terminology – the manifested matter due to perception is called Maya.

The different vibrations, forces and celestial phenomena became different Gods (Devtas and Devis) and their attributes. The consciousness behind the creation is Brahman and it pervades what has manifested as the universe - different objects and energies and bodies and pervades it. It is the seed from the entire creation has burst forth and unto which it dissolves. Maharishi Patanjali says similarly that God is omniscient – it is all knowing and the source of all knowledge. There is nothing beyond God.

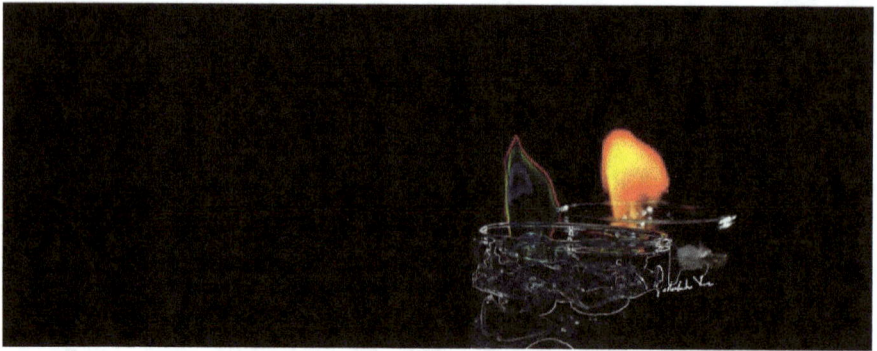

1.26

THE MASTER

स पूर्वेषाम् अपि गुरुः कालेनानवच्छेदात् ॥
pūrveṣām api guruḥ kālenānavacchedāt ॥
(Sa purveshaam api Guru, kaalena Anvcchedaat)

God is timeless and is the Guru of the earliest Gurus.

"A Guru's very existence in life grants you the impossible." - Sri Sri Ravi Shankar

The importance of the Master is finally mentioned by Maharishi Patanjali in this sutra. After giving us the aim of Yoga, he finally tells the aspirant that each Saint and Yogi who achieved success on this path had a Master, a guide.

The earliest of the Masters, who are said to have been revealed this knowledge in deep states of meditation, their Guru was the Divine Consciousness, God. In Bhagavad Gita, Lord Krishna tells Arjuna:

श्री भगवानुवाच ।
इमं विवस्वते योगं प्रोक्तवानहमव्ययम् । विवस्वान्मनवे प्राह मनुरिक्ष्वाकवेऽब्रवीत् ॥ ४.१

Lord Krishna said: I taught this eternal science of Yoga to the Sun God Vivasvan, who imparted it to Manu; Manu in-turn taught it to

Ikshvaku. (Chapter 4, Verse 1)

Lord Krishna is telling Arjuna that He is eternal, and the Guru of all Gurus. Similarly, Maharishi Patanjali is telling God is timeless, omnipresent and the Master of all the masters. A Guru understands the need of the student and all he wants is for the student to succeed. The Guru Element is necessary to achieve success. The aspirant here must understand the need of a Guru, and must place his complete faith in him, for the last step can be climbed only by the Grace of the Master.

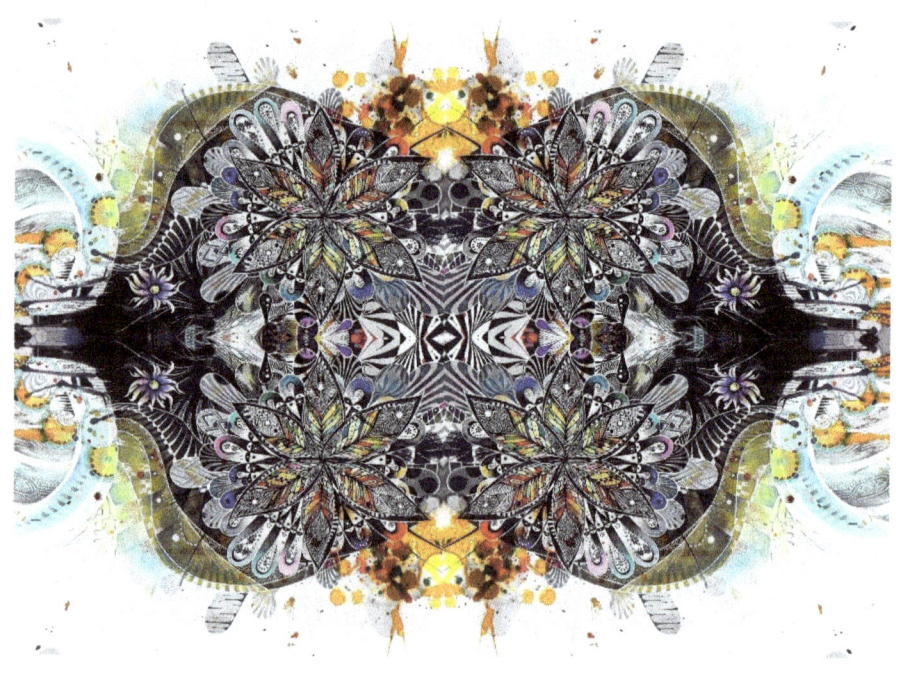

1.27

SOUND OF GOD

तस्य वाचकः प्रणवः ॥
tasya vācakaḥ praṇavaḥ ॥
(Tasya Vaachaka Pranava)

The sound form of God is Pranav.

Every religion has given a sacred sound: Hinduism has OM, Islam has Ameen, Christianity and Judaism have Amen, and Sikhism has Ik-Omkar. It is no coincidence that all these sounds are so similar to each other even though they originated thousands of miles and millennia away from each other.

Many researches have conducted to study the effect of sound on body. The more healing the sound is, the more symmetrical are the water crystals that form. Since the human body is more than 60% water, sound directly impacts the body-mind complex.

Pranav simply means a sacred sound. The rustling of the leaves in a gentle breeze, the waves lapping at the shore, a rivulet chiming as it moves through the woods, the cracking of fire on a cold winter day - the sound of breath and life itself: the entire cosmos is just vibrations.

The sound of pure consciousness is OM. Pranav also means OM. AUM is made up of three syllables and represents the three energies of the universe – Creative (Generation), Maintaining (Operation), and Transformative (Destruction). This cycle of the universe is perpetual. Every day the Sun rises (Generation), gives energy and life to all (Maintenance) and then sets (Destruction) to regenerate the next day.

It also represents the three states of mind – Awakened, Sleeping, and Dreaming. It represents the Trigunas – Sattva, Rajas, and Tamas.

The fourth part of AUM is Silence which represents the state beyond the three states. God encompasses all the energies, and is beyond it. All the states of the mind are in the realm of Brahman, but Brahman is also beyond - it cannot be grasped by the intellect or the ego – it is the transcendental state. The one who rises above the influence of the Trigunas experiences Brahman. Sri Sri Ravi Shankar says that the purpose of all words and sounds is to bring a contented Silence in the mind – words and sounds that create disturbance are to be dropped.

OM is the journey from Sound to Silence. There is a beautiful guided meditation that you can do to experience this journey.
https://www.youtube.com/watch?v=8nUzsR5HZYo

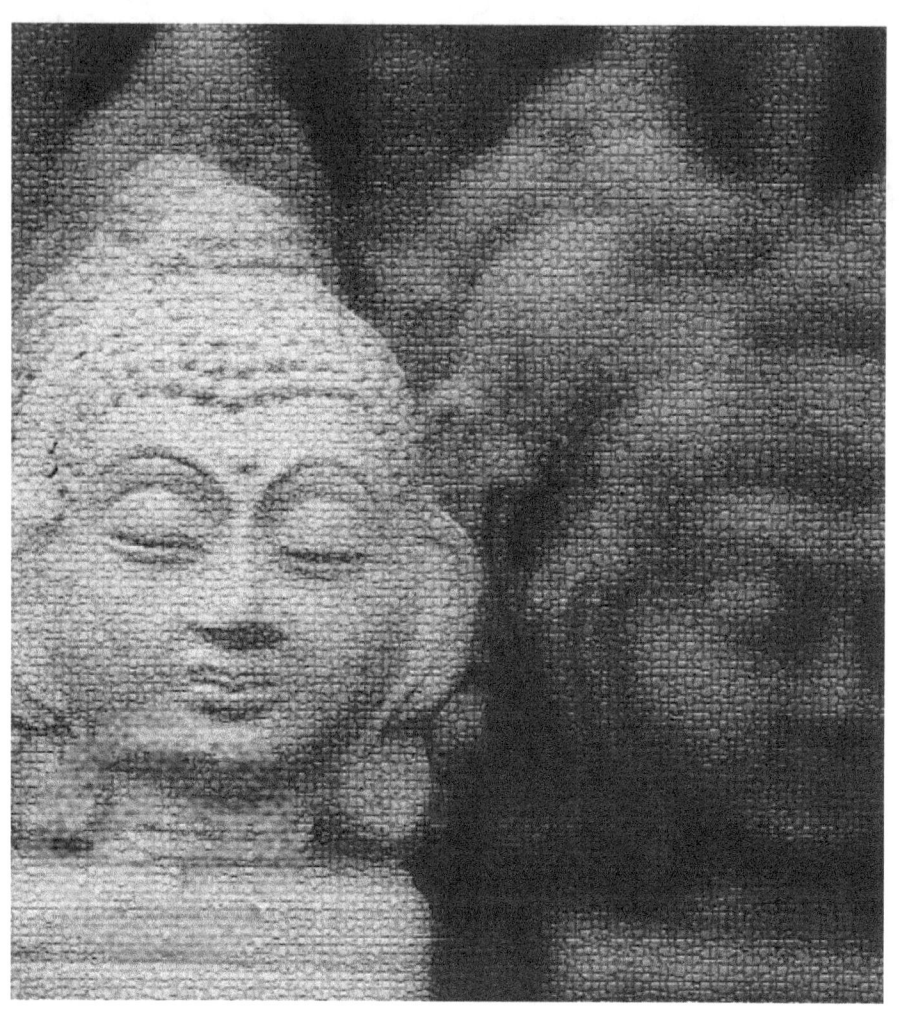

1.28

THE SECRET OF MANTRA

तज्जपस्तदर्थभावनम् ॥
Tajjapastadarthabhāvanam ॥
(Tat japa, Tat artha Bhavana)

Repetition of That (AUM) illumines its essence in our Being.

"A mantra when constantly repeated awakens the consciousness." - Swami Sivananda

An average person that sets out to do any task usually has his mind wandering at a few places while doing the task. The result is poor understanding, a scattered mind, and a loss of efficacy. There is a lack of awareness in the present moment and much that could be perceived is lost. No matter where the mind stays, experience can only take place in the present moment and that is what actually brings change. Any task done mechanically loses a lot of potency. The mind has to work in tandem with the body and vice versa to achieve a state of mind that flows. As Jordan Peterson mentions in his book '12 Rules for Life', when one is completely engrossed in the work one is doing such that even the flow of time is unnoticeable, that is when life reveals itself and one steps from the known into the unknown. It is at this juncture when the most profound meaning well up from the depths of our own very being. This is aligned with the idea that the greatest knowledge is which comes from within and not without, Brahman or God can only be experienced. Speeches, discourses, books, and commentaries – these all can provide knowledge, create interest, and inspire a person to explore the dimension of higher consciousness. But knowledge is not experience, and that which is not in experience is not transformational. Scholars can never reach the highest states of consciousness with their analysis and debates because even logic has limitations. There are things that cannot be rationalized.

It is hard to dive into the unmanifest. Since the manifest arises from the unmanifest, we can use it as well. That manifest form is OM. The emotion behind this sound makes a difference. A desire to realize the Brahman within makes it more potent. Reciting the Mantra with awareness and devotion, with humility and intensity, can take us into Samadhi where the essence of the Mantra is revealed from within.

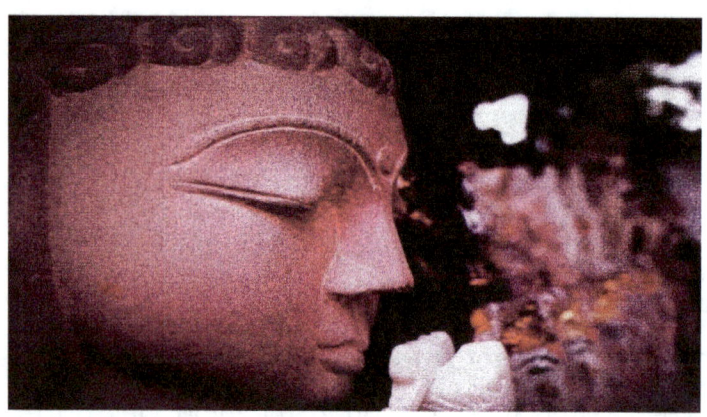

1.29

THE POWER OF MANTRA

ततः प्रत्यक्चेतनाधिगमोऽप्यन्तरायाभावश्च ॥
tataḥ pratyakcetanādhigamo'pyantarāyābhāvaśca ॥
(tatah Pratyak-chetna-adhigama, api Antaraaya-abhava cha)

That (recitation of AUM) reveals the true inner Consciousness; and also removes all obstacles.

> "Mantra is God. God Himself is the Mantra."
> -Swami Chidananda

We all experience doubts, sadness, misery, and frustration that shakes us from our center. In fact, even happiness and joy often shake us from our center. There are a lot of days we question the meaning and purpose of everything in our lives. People, environment, and circumstances affect the mind no matter how strong we are. It is the nature of the world and the mind. Some aspirants interpret the knowledge of the scriptures poorly; they expect to never go through another fluctuation of the mind ever again once they start practicing some technique. Such people may have started the technique for this end only – they are escapists. There is no escape – the only way is through.

One becomes centered when one goes through all kinds of experiences (pleasurable and painful) and gradually learns to respond, and not react, externally, and keep the peace intact within.

The method of reciting OM is not only for those who cannot put effort to attain success on this path, it is also for those who are putting their intense desire and effort into it. The Japa (recitation) of the mantra removes obstacles that may arise in the path of Yoga.

A Mantra roughly translated also means 'That which takes the Mind Beyond.' A Mantra is like a vehicle which carries the mind across all the Vrittis. It purifies it of impressions and concepts and helps it achieve clarity. It should be incorporated by everyone in their Sadhana.

1.30

THE CHALLENGE

व्याधिस्त्यानसंशयप्रमादालस्याविरतिभ्रान्तिदर्शनालब्धभूमिकत्वानवस्थितत्वानि
चित्तविक्षेपास्तेऽन्तरायाः ॥

vyādhistyānasaṁśayapramādālasyāviratibhrāntidarśanālabdha-
bhūmikatvānavasthitatvāni cittavikṣepāste'ntarāyāḥ ॥

(Vyaadhi Styaana Samshaya Pramaada Aalasya Avirati
Bhranti-darshana Alabdha-bhumikatva Anavasthi-tatvaani, Chitta vikshepa te
antaraaya)

Disease, mental illness, doubt, carelessness, laziness, sensory abuse, false perception, failing to attain progress in practice, and inability to maintain the state of practice – these obstacles arise in the consciousness.

Disease and health, like circumstances, are rooted in thought." - James Allen

A wise man once said, "The first step to solve a problem is to accept there is a problem." The path to success is not without its fair share of impediments. In the spiritual path of Yoga, all the hindrances are internal – no one can be blamed, but also that means they all can be taken care of by oneself if one is courageous enough to take responsibility. All the obstacles that may block someone from achieving growth on the path have been mentioned here –

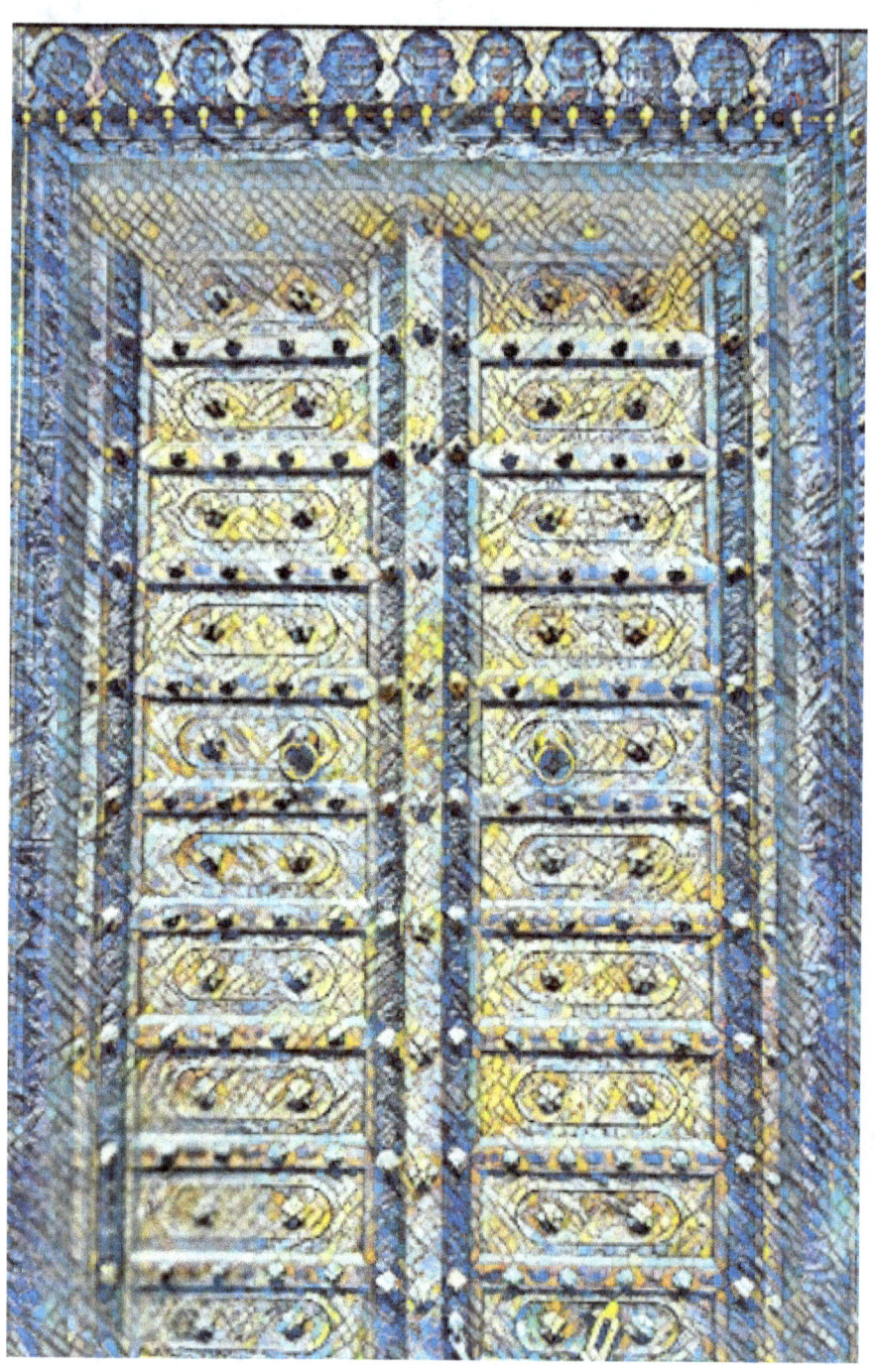

1. Vyadhi – disease of the body.
2. Styana – disease of the mind.
3. Samshaya – doubt

Doubt is of 3 types:
- Doubt on the Self – A lot of people feel depreciating oneself is a virtuous quality. There is a difference being modest and considering oneself worthless. Such people underestimate themselves at every stage, get comfortable with failure, and consequently, misery and resentment. Success of any venture takes responsibility. The Sadhakas tend to undermine their worth – they would have doubts over whether they are even worth the knowledge they have received, or if a "sinful" person like them would ever deserve peace and bliss. This doubt brings lack of effort because effort seems fruitless and when the lack of effort does cause failure, it only strengthens the doubt that actually resulted in it.

- Doubt on the Master – the disciple doubts the Guru or may even wonder if he is the correct person to be a Guru. In the current age where there have been so many incidents of people exploiting the faith of people for their personal pleasures and goals, a lot of people are repulsed by the idea of a spiritual Guru.

- Doubt on the Technique - one can find out information about different saints easily and the different techniques they are offering. If the faith is not strong, some people embark on a journey of a spiritual window shopping – they go to different places, and try to see what is being offered without taking anything with humility and gratitude.

4. Pramada – Carelessness. This obstacle is the most commonly observed obstacle by people in others. To observe it in oneself, a degree of self-awareness is required. Non-smokers wonder why people smoke even when the cigarette pack itself says smoking causes cancer. Doctors are one of the highest spending groups on liquor. Households are filled with diabetic people who will not give up sweets. And Pramada is not just doing what one ought to not do, it is also not-doing what one ought to do. A student not studying even as exams approach is in Pramada. Procrastination falls under Pramada. Pramada can be understood as not taking responsibility for one's life. Responsibility gives us choice in every situation, and carelessness takes away the choice.

5. Alasya – Lethargy/Laziness.

6. Avirati – Overindulgence in Senses. The mind is looking for the infinite, and the senses have a limited capacity of deriving pleasure from sensory objects. But if someone has no higher goal in life other than enjoying the sensory pleasures, it slowly erodes the intellect, motivation and desire for something higher and brings dullness and inertia. - The senses are always directed outwards, but creativity and innovation can be nurtured by spending time with oneself in silence. Avirati ends in loss of the

ability to enjoy even the sensory objects for there is a limit to how much pleasure senses can derive.

7. BhrantiDarshana – Delusion. Getting stuck in fantasies of achieving supernatural abilities (siddhis) by doing practices, and developing unfounded fears and phobias to protect oneself is BhrantiDarshana.

8. AlabdhaBhumikatva – inability to achieve any kind of success in Sadhana. This can damage the faith of the practitioner and breed doubt and dullness.

9. AnavasthiTatva – being unable to maintain success of Sadhana.

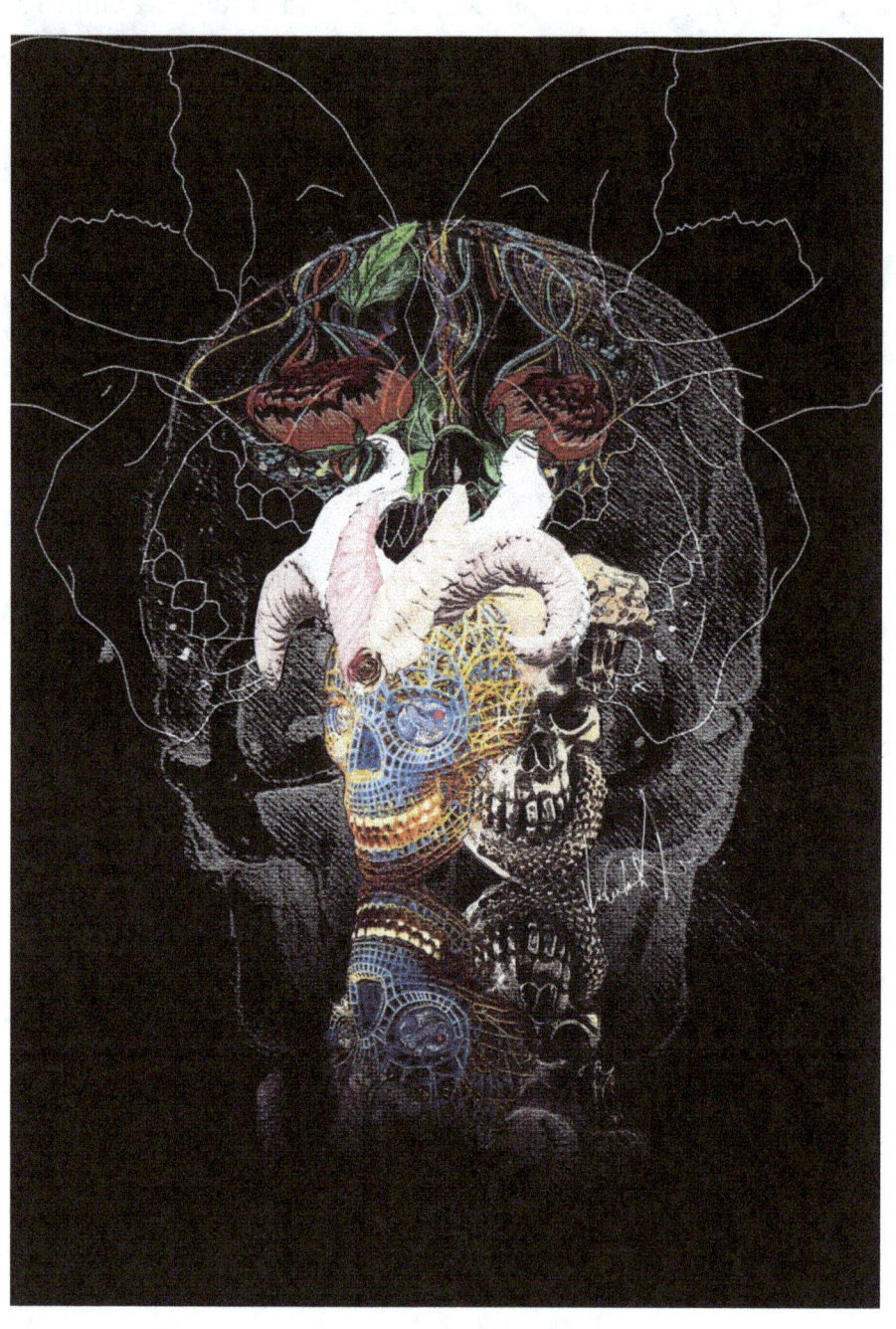

1.31

WATCH OUT FOR THE SIGNS

दुःखदौर्मनस्याङ्गमेजयत्वश्वासप्रश्वासा विक्षेपसहभुवः ॥
duḥkhadaurmanasyāṅgamejayatvaśvāsapraśvāsā
vikṣepasahabhuvaḥ ॥
(Dukha Daurmanasya Angame-jayatva Shvaasa-prashvaasa-vikshepa Saha-bhuva)

Grief, Resentment, Lack of control over body, and Irregular breathing, are the symptoms that one is facing a challenge on his path.

"The only way we can change the way we feel is by becoming aware of our inner experience and learning to befriend what is going inside ourselves."
- Bessel van der Kolk

Everyone faces one or more of the nine obstacles listed in the previous sutra on their spiritual or material path. Many a times, for many of us, it becomes difficult to recognize we are going through a block. Having a signpost can help.

• **Dukha** – Grief/Sadness: We all have to go through tough times. Failure, loss, disease, injury, and much more. Grief and sadness are as solid as the next rock that you will kick in frustration. One cannot get rid of these natural emotions that everyone has a fair share of in their life. But we should not be stuck in these emotions. There is something that needs to be changed if that is the case. Maybe it is the job, or our toxic relationships, or our family/friends, or our own insecurities that are making us miserable all the time.

• **Dourmanasya** – Bitterness: We all have fantasized about revenge in one form of the other – Oh, I should have said this in reply to his insult, I should have humiliated her that one time when I had the chance, I wish he had never shown up in my life, etc. We are unable to stop blaming people and God. Holding on to grudges and the bitterness is Hell. The mind starts spouting insecurities. Anger becomes a permanent tenant. Negativity clouds the brain. Forgiveness is a virtue of the brave. Yes, people do things that hurt, that destroy and that cause immense pain and agony. One can physically move away from them, if possible, but removing them from mind takes forgiveness. What they did was their choice, but allowing them to still destroy you while they are not there is ours. We need to forgive people and God for our sake. Focusing on the positive things in life, expressing gratitude, standing up for yourself and being a responsible human being goes a long, long way in keeping the bitterness away.

• **Angamejayatva** – Lack of Control over the Body: The body is a tool as well as an instrument. If it listens to the mind and helps you fulfil the tasks you set out to do, it is a good tool. For that, it must be kept disease free, healthy, and fit. The state of the body tells the state of the mind. If the body is unable to take any kind of hard work, or if it refuses to get up and work and feels sleepy all the time resulting in anxiety and apprehensions, then it is a poor tool and an instrument which tells us the body and mind are not in sync.

Fear, anxiety, jealousy, and other undesirable emotions have a physiological effect – the breath becomes shallow, the heart speeds up, the immune system becomes weak, the blood pressure fluctuates, the eyes fail to focus, the legs stumble over each other, and the hands are unable to grasp anything. The body fails to listen to you. Senses frantically try to gather some information that might quell the storm that is raging in the mind. We binge on music, Netflix and e-commerce sites. Something is wrong, and we must not be afraid of asking for help.

- **Shvasa-prashavasa Vikshepa** – Irregular Breathing: The breath is the mirror of the mind. There is a very interesting experiment you could do with yourself. Sit comfortably where no one will disturb you for a few minutes.

Try different breathing patterns. Hold your breath for some time and see what emotions arise. Then breathe fast and shallow and observe. Breathe fast and deep and observe. Breathe loudly and observe. Breathe gently and deeply and observe. You may not be able to observe your emotions the first time you attempt this. Some Yogic practices like Pranayama and Meditation may help you increase your awareness, or you can attempt this repeatedly over a few days and try to observe. You will understand why irregular breathing is a symptom of a disturbed mind.

It is quite possible that pranayama and meditation may also result in these symptoms. Many people experience grief in their meditations, or their breathing becomes strained and irregular during practicing Pranayama. It is a temporary state caused due elimination of the toxin. The impressions that were hiding in the subconscious mind surface and many years of pent-up emotions and desires cause people to cry and scream and laugh hysterically. Doubts and apprehensions which surface during the practices are mostly issues that we have been brushing under the carpet and need to address. These symptoms are easily noticed. They are not to be ignored because that really does not solve anything.

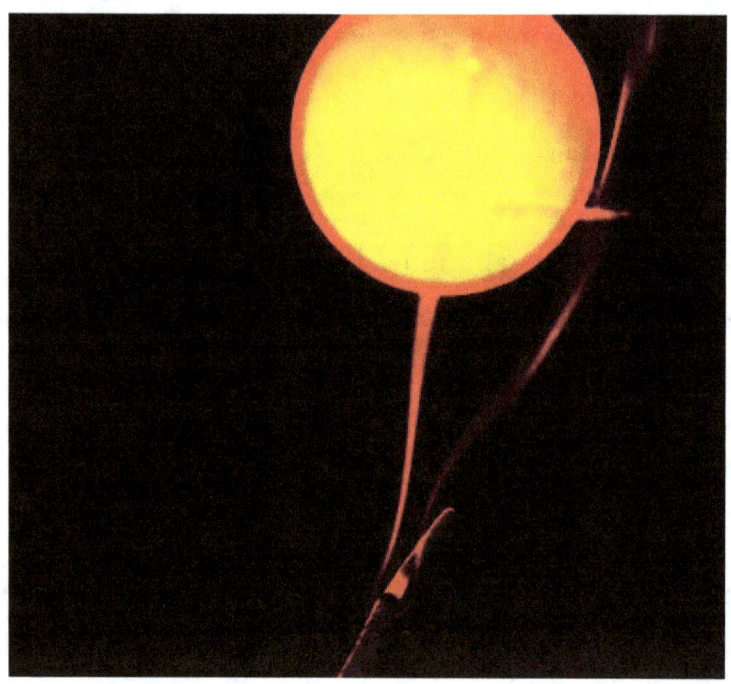

1.32

ONE THING TO RULE THEM ALL

तत्प्रतिषेधार्थमेकतत्त्वाभ्यासः ॥
tatpratiṣedhārthamekatattvābhyāsaḥ ॥
(tat Pratished-artham, Ek-tattva-abhyaasa)

To overcome all the difficulties on the path,
Focus and Aim all your energy on a
Single objective/technique.

"Focus and Simplicity – once you get there, you can move mountains." - Steve Jobs

Remember the Ring Wraiths from the Lord of the Rings? The undead Nine Kings of Men cursed to find the Ring of Sauron for ever? No matter where the ring bearer went, they always found him. No place was safe – neither a cave in the coldest mountain, nor the dungeons deep in the ground, and nor the strongest fortress of men. The Wraiths had only one thought in their enslaved minds – The Ring. This focus, the one-pointedness made them overcome any terrain, any magic, and all types of battles.

One can learn an important lesson from these characters, one which Maharishi Patanjali is also reiterating in this sutra. All the people who have achieved extra-ordinary results in their fields have this characteristic – one pointedness. They become blind to everything but their aim, and their will becomes sharp as a sword, able to cut through the most daunting challenges.

If we want success in a big endeavour, then we must put all our energies in that endeavour. We do not have to start doing new things in most of the cases, we just have to stop doing things that are not helping us achieve our target. There are a lot of activities we do in our day that have absolutely no impact on taking us closer to our goal.

We have to make a choice - to choose one technique that suits us the best, and focus all our energy into it. The complexity of the technique is insignificant. If one is practicing Mantra Yoga, chant one mantra. Do not go on changing the Mantra at a whim or under influence. The Mantra is usually received from the Guru, which makes it infinitely potent.

A Master would never change the Mantra if you have already received one from another saint. If you are using a symbol for meditation, choose and stick with one symbol. The consciousness has to work from scratch if you keep on changing the tool you are using. The mind gets scattered and that is not conducive to success. This one-pointedness and focus will invariably bring success in the Yogic Path as well other endeavours as well.

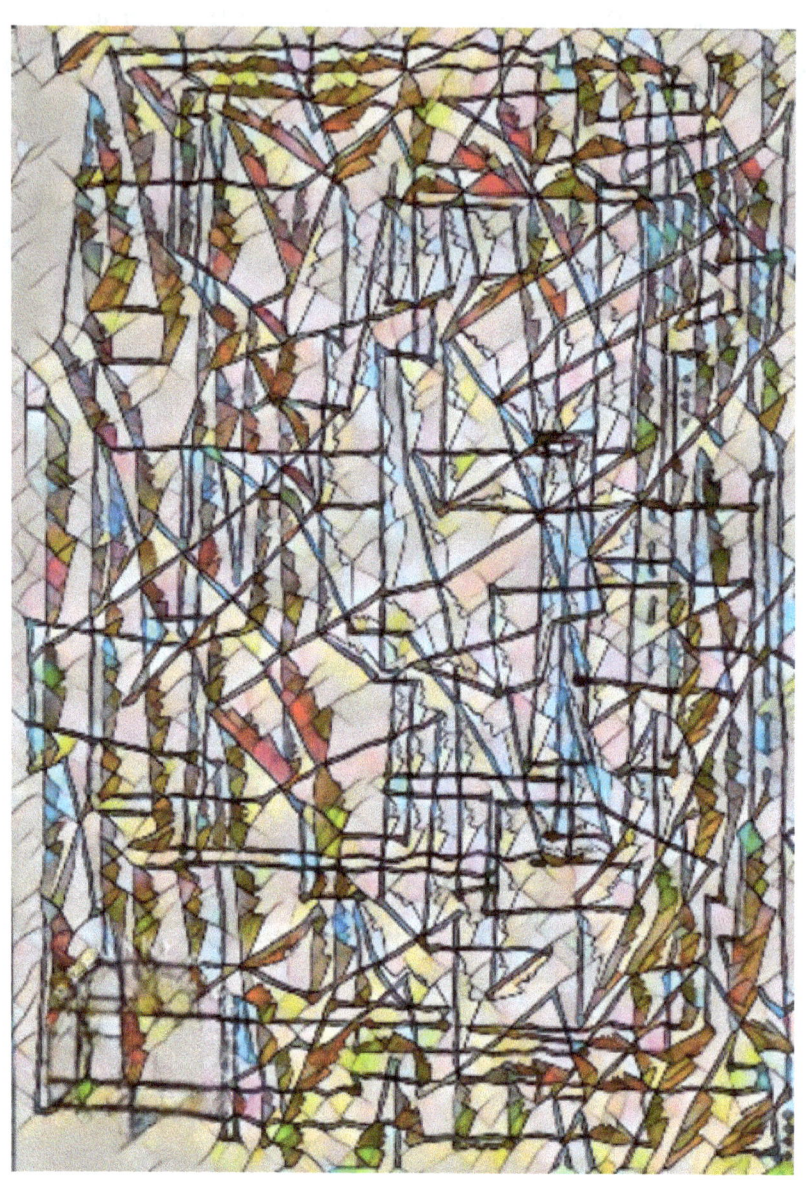

1.33

PEOPLE PEOPLE EVERYWHERE

मैत्रीकरुणामुदितोपेक्षाणां सुखदुःखपुण्यापुण्यविषयाणां भावनातश्चित्तप्रसादनम् ॥
maitrīkaruṇāmuditopekṣāṇāṁ sukhaduḥkha-
puṇyāpuṇyaviṣayāṇāṁ bhāvanātaścittaprasādanam ॥
(Maitri Karunaa Muditaa Upekshanaam, Sukha Dukha Punya Apunya vishyanaam, Bhaavna Chitta-Prasaada)

By cultivating an attitude of Friendliness towards the happy, Compassion towards the miserable, Delight towards the virtuous, and Indifference towards the unrighteous; one can attain peace of mind and overcome the obstacles.

"Hell is other people." - Jean Paul Satre

Human Beings are social animals, much dependent on the societal structure to grow, develop and turn into adults who help to make the world better. Our moods and our attitude towards people make a great deal of our state of mind. We all encounter people up to no good, out to disrupt plans and cause havoc because that is who they are. Many people are hurtful. Many are committed to morally compromised acts, and many who have made misery their identity and use that misery to pull others down too.

There are people who are successful and then there are those who are jovial and charming. It is not what people do, what how we react to what people do that we can control.

In this sutra, Maharishi Patanjali gives the secret to dealing with people in our lives. People are found in broadly 4 states of being:
- Happy
- Miserable
- Engaged in Righteous acts
- Engaged in Unrighteous acts

Any person can be in these different states at different points of time. There are some qualities of our family members that are endearing, and some utterly annoying. You like your friend's kindness, and but his stubbornness makes you want to punch him. And some cases are not so simple. Even if we do not want to, sometimes jealousy arises when someone tastes success. We get into conflict with ourselves, arguing that this is not who we are. We usually create a distance from someone we are jealous of. We are mostly full of contempt for those who have no moral compass. We are stuck in both "good" and "bad", letting the mind run in one direction or the other. If we can control our reaction to the acts and states of being of other people, we can keep our mind peaceful, not get distracted and continue towards our goal.

Friendly towards the happy – You are a real friend if you are happy when the friend achieves something and is happy. You do not try to upstage him, bring him down or become resentful. It can be practiced the other way around to keep the mind peaceful. For all those that are happy and successful, have a friendly attitude towards them. Now, the attitude is in the mind. You may not actually be friends with such people, but you can train yourself to be happy for them, to appreciate them, and also to take inspiration from them. This keeps the mind on a positive track. It takes some practice to be happy for the successful for resentment is very easy nowadays. Once you are happy for them, their success does not trouble you, and it does not dwarf your happiness in any way. You do not grovel in self-pity even if things are not as fortunate for you. In fact, it boosts your happiness further. This allows you to learn good things from them and yourself become happier and more successful.

Compassion for the Miserable – Misery is part of life, and more often than not, there is something that we can do about it if we are really looking to get out of it. On the other hand, it is very easy to build an identity around our misery, to make it an excuse for our failures, vices, and shortcomings. We make friends with people just so that we would have an ear to tell how unfair the world has been to us. It is not that misery is to be condescended – it is not to be glorified. We must not pity the miserable, we must be compassionate towards them. A compassionate mother of an ill child does not tell her son that disease is wrong in affecting him – she teaches him to be stronger and how to take care of himself. If you tell a miserable person that he has absolutely no hand in bringing the misery on himself (which is not true in most cases), we strip that person of his power to set things right. Many people do not want to get out of misery because it is a free-pass card. People will excuse them. They do not know what they will do if they were not miserable. There is no obligation to associate with such people. Be compassionate for them, help them if you can but be away from them if they are not ready to get better. Protect your mind at all costs.

Delighting in the Righteous – It takes strength to be stand beside someone who has integrity of character and the courage to do what needs to be done without complaints. Such people make us very self-aware of our own weaknesses, our own temptations to which we frequently give in and these are not good emotions. We become angry, and instead of truly understanding that we are angry at ourselves, we project the anger on the virtuous people and more often than not, we label them as arrogant. When such labels enter the mind, we become cynical, and cannot believe anyone do good without having an ulterior motive. It is a poor state of mind which causes a lot of pain. The mind wants to feel positive, and it tries to repeat things which made it feel positive. Delighting in the acts of the righteous trains the mind to be happy in virtuous acts (use your understanding to see what you categorize as righteous or unrighteous). We start emulating such acts ourself. We start developing a better personality. In the face of the virtuous, we stand tall, and use it as an opportunity to be virtuous as well.

Indifferent towards the unrighteousness – This might be the most difficult thing to do. Unrighteousness does not mean only wrong acts. It means anything you may not approve of or dislike. There may be someone you find stupid. Once you label them as stupid, all you can perceive is the label. They stop being a complex human being for you. Your perception is destroyed. Same goes for people you dislike. Every time you encounter them, all you can feel is your dislike, and you view every act and listen to every word of their speech with disdain even if they are speaking something that might be beneficial – for you or someone else. It is very easy to feel smug. It then becomes very easy to turn people into labels. It is a violent process if seen objectively – a person is destroyed and made into a word. View people as people. So many people are engaged in wrongful acts too. They cannot be at peace because their conscience will not let them at sleep. Your disdain for such people does not let you be at peace – both good and bad are not at peace. Indifference does not mean you do not do anything to prevent wrongful acts. It just means you do not let it cloud your consciousness; you do not let it affect your core.

Educate and let go.

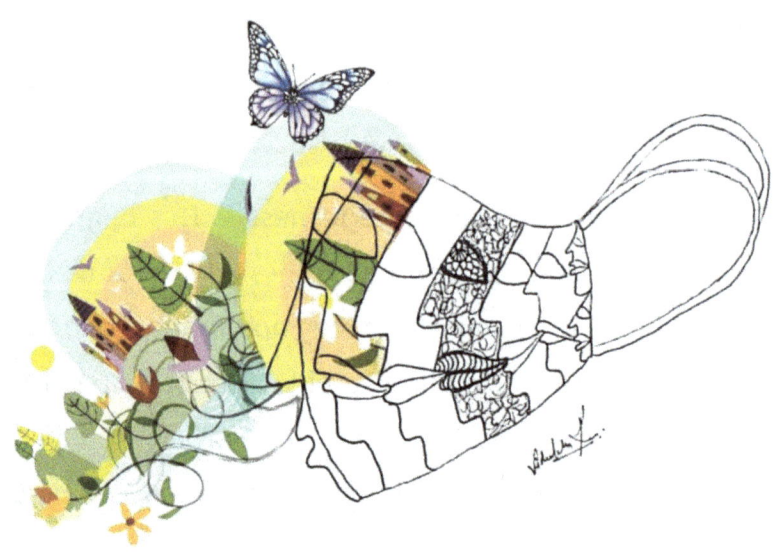

1.34

MIND YOUR BREATH

प्रच्छर्दनविधारणाभ्यां वा प्राणस्य ॥
pracchardanavidhāraṇābhyāṁ vā prāṇasya ॥
(Pracchardana-vidharnaabhyam vaa Pranasya)

or by Changing the pattern of the breath
→ holding the breath out
(One can bring the mind under control and keep it peaceful).

"Breath is the biggest secret nature has put in you."
- Sri Sri Ravi Shankar

An experiment was conducted at the Menninger Foundation, USA on Swami Nadabrahmananda Saraswati, an Indian Classical Musician who had perfected the science of Thaan. He became a disciple of Swami Sivananda Saraswati in his later years. The experiment intended to verify his claim that he could stay without breathing for long periods of time.

He was placed in an airtight chamber, with his nose and ears blocked and body smeared with wax. He had his Tabla with him. An alive monkey and a burning candle were placed in similar chambers. After 3 minutes, the candle flamed out, and after another 10 minutes, the monkey fell unconscious, but Swamiji continued playing the Tabla. There was a coin placed on the top of his shaved head which kept bobbing up and down.

He played the Tabla for 40 minutes without breathing. He explained that he controlled the flow of Prana inside his body and one lives as long as Prana exists even if one is not breathing.

The Pranic Body envelopes the physical body and it is responsible for all functions of the body. Breath is the bridge between the Gross/Physical Body and Pranic Body. Through the ages, Pranayama has been one of the fundamental parts of the Yogic practices. Enlightened Masters have taught various breathing techniques to control the Prana and hence control the mind. The Yogic texts say there are 72000 nadis or pranic channels in the subtle body through which Prana flows. One Prana assumes different forms in different parts of the body to fulfil different functions. If the Prana flows unobstructed, the body-mind complex stays healthy.

Some of the most popular Pranayama in current times are Nadi Shodhan Pranayama, Kapal Bhati Pranayama, Ujjayi Pranayama,

Bhastrika Pranayama, and Bhramari Pranayama. The above sutra explains one of the techniques of Pranayama (Bahir Kumbhaka – holding the breath outside), but it essentially refers to the connection between mind, prana and breath. The breath can be understood as gross form of Prana, which everyone can work with to develop control over the subtle Prana.

The breath is to the mind what string is to a kite. It is the breath which needs to be controlled to perfect any skill - music, sports, martial arts, academics, etc. The breath is the secret to a lively life.

You can do a small experiment to confirm this – take long deep breaths (both inhalation and exhalation) in a relaxed manner and see the state of your mind. Then, take hurried breaths, as if you are scared. The pattern of the breath immediately affects the state of the mind. The cause and effect are intertwined – the state of the mind affects the breath but we are usually too caught up with the mind to notice it – the state of the breath affects the mind. If we become a little aware, and develop control over the mind, we can also handle the thoughts better.

Learning a Pranayama from a Master and practicing it diligently can bring supernatural awareness in the mind. One can control which thought stays and which one passes, and build laser like focus. It is one of the most powerful methods to be disease free physically, emotionally and mentally, achieve great things in life and ascend to higher states of living.

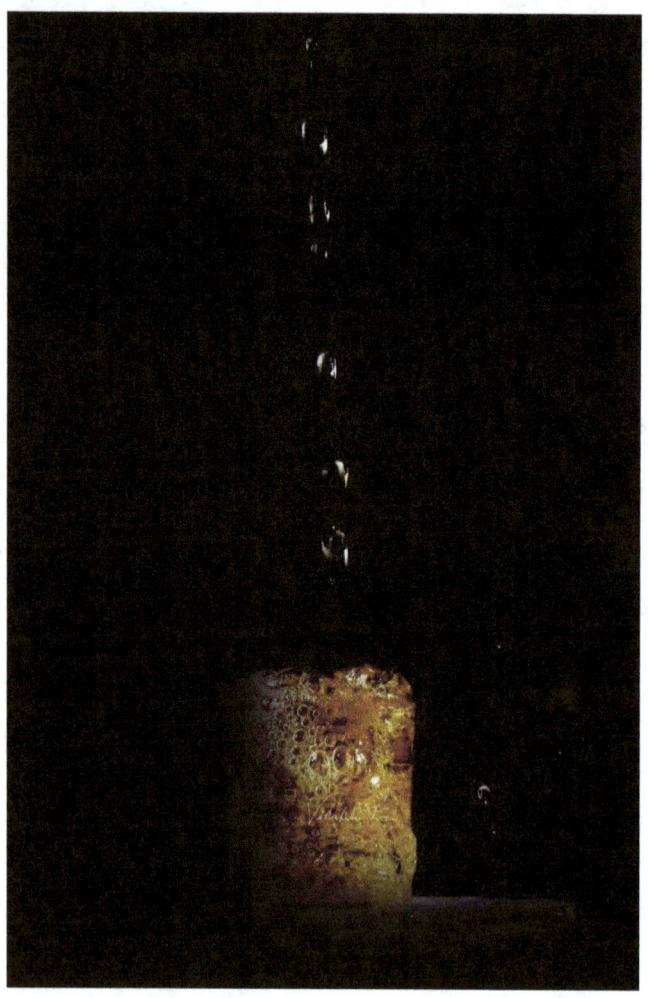

1.35

THE REAL-SURREAL CONNECTIONS

विषयवती वा प्रवृत्तिरुत्पन्ना मनसः स्थितिनिबन्धिनी ॥
viṣayavatī vā pravṛttirutpannā manasaḥ sthitinibandhinī ॥
(Vishayavati vaa pravritti utpanna, Manasa sthiti nibandhini)

Or else, the mind can be stabilised by arresting it in a sensory experience/object.

"Nothing can satisfy the soul but the senses, and nothing can satisfy the senses but the soul."
- Oscar Wilde, The Picture of Dorian Gray

Take a minute and mentally picture the first 15 minutes after you wake up every day. What is it like? Waking up to an alarm(s), looking at your phone, stretching your body, freshening up. The rest of the day is spent observing, speaking, listening, tasting and touching. After crashing to sleep (for many of us, it happens after our phone makes a dent in the face), the senses do not let you be even in your sleep – you dream.

We are a generation with all forms of sensory objects at instant disposal. We can work from our homes, even on our phones, and entertain ourselves to all kinds of media anywhere, anytime. Where is the opportunity to be without a sensory object in our mental experience? It is not possible for most of us to simply give up all sensory object even for 20 minutes a day.

In this sutra, the beauty of Yoga as a path of acceptance and growth is revealed. Instead of prophesying certain doom for those who cannot do without their sensory objects, a way is given to use the sensory object itself for stabilizing the mind from which it may start on the path of disassociating with the vrittis. There are many techniques that use the sensory object for steadying the mind.

One of them is Trataka. In Trataka, an object is chosen (usually a candle flame) for the eyes to gaze at without blinking for as long as possible. The practice can be performed for as short a time period as 30 seconds – it depends on how long can a person gaze unblinkingly without feeling strain in their eyes. With time and practice, a person may be able to hold the gaze for 30 minutes. This is Bahir Trataka (external Trataka). The goal of the practice is to be able to view the object on the mental screen with eyes closed – Antar Trataka (internal Trataka). It Is thus advised not to change the object once it is chosen, otherwise the mind is not able to grasp onto the object and visualize it.

Bringing the mind under control using sound is a common practice in many religions. Kirtan and Satsang are a common occurrence in temples and ashrams around the world. Usually in bhajans, only one word is repeated. It slowly gathers the mind and allows it to settle. The mind slowly dissolves into the word and moves into transcendental state of awareness. There are other techniques also involving the sense of touch and taste, but they are advanced and must be learned from a Master.

1.36

THERE IS A LIGHT THAT NEVER GOES OUT

विशोका वा ज्योतिष्मती ॥
viśokā vā jyotiṣmatī ॥
(Vishoka vaa Jyotishmati)

In the sorrowless state, by attuning the mind to the illumination within (one can control the mind).

"There is a light that never goes out."
- The Smiths, The Queen Is Dead

Sadness and misery seem to take out energy from us. Research shows that people who are sad, or clinically depressed may tend to sleep more. When we are happy, we feel enthusiastic and dynamic. We feel ready to do anything. In this state, when we are happy and cheerful, stabilizing the mind is easy. If we can hold this state for longer and longer periods of time, the mind can come under control, and conversely, as the mind stabilizes, we will be more peaceful and cheerful.

There are thoughts itself which are illuminating – they bring Sattvik happiness – happiness that is untainted and blissful. The thought is not supposed to provide any answers or insights, the thought simply removes all that is false. This illumination clears the intellect and the memory from deep set patterns in the unconscious mind.

Ramana Maharishi, a great saint from South India who - lived in the 20th century, said that the path of self-enquiry, sitting with the thought of "Who am I" will set one free.

Another dimension is focusing on the sensory objects within. The sensory objects without, no matter how subtle, are gross in nature. If we keep on listening to music outside, we will never sit in silence and try to attune to the music within. If we keep on looking at the candle flame, we will never close our eyes and see the flame burning within.

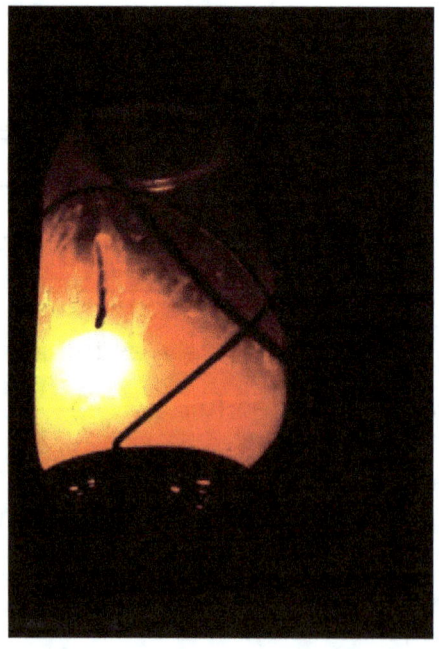

All that is without is within, says the Shiva Samhita. This sutra follows the same theme. Yogic texts talk about visualizing light at one of two locations – in the center of the chest (the Anahata Chakra), or the center of the head, in between the eyebrows (the Ajna Chakra).

With time and regular practice, the practitioner is able to visualize the light and the mind progresses inwards at a great speed, dropping its patterns and associations. Distractions, and uncontrolled thoughts fall off. Another sensory object is the Anahat Naad – the unstruck sound that is sound of the soul. Laya Yoga expounds on attaining Liberation by tuning into the Anahat Naad.

The mental fortitude and clarity of intellect and memory required to be able to focus on the sensory object within, or a particular thought within is the purpose of techniques like Trataka. All other techniques discussed before also aim to refine the memory and remove learned and conditioned patterns which in fact have no foundation, and are not the basis of how to live life.

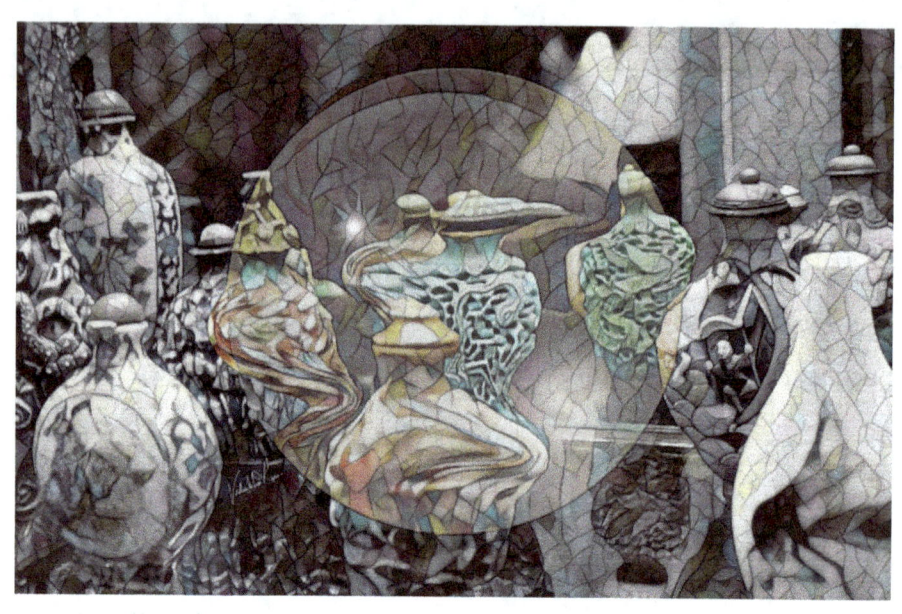

1.37

BE LIKE WATER MY FRIEND

वीतरागविषयं वा चित्तम् ॥
vītarāgaviṣayaṁ vā cittam ॥
(Vita Raaga Vishyam vaa Chitta)

By remembering the One who is devoid of cravings (the mind can be made steady).

"Mind is like water – it becomes the thought you engage in."
- Sri Sri Ravi Shankar, An Intimate Note to the Sincere Seeker

Go and ask a 5th grader about the five elements the body is made up of – Earth, Water, Fire, Air and Space/Ether. Go to the greatest scientists, biochemists, neuroscientists in the world and ask them what elements is the mind made of, or if it even exists and see if you get a conclusive answer.

There is no experiment yet to verify the existence of consciousness. The only proof is the claim that I have a mind, but the individual claim is not a concrete proof in the field of science. What the mind is, and from where it generates its thoughts and moods is debatable for modern science. It is a difficult topic to express for the ancient science and philosophy as well, but it does a better job in providing insights of its workings and how to handle it.

Swami Vivekananda said, "We are what our thoughts have made us; so, take care about what you think." In my childhood, I used to get angry at my friends frequently. I would complain to my mother about their actions and how they irritate me. My mother used to tell me that if I keep thinking about them, I would also start doing the things I do not like. As I grew up, I have noticed this occurrence – I have noticed the qualities of the people I think about to manifest in me. It is very subtle, it is very minute, but it happens. You can experiment with yourself.

Think about a person who has a short temper and shouts for no reason. Your head will tense up and you may even feel a little angry yourself. Now, think about a person who loves you very much – can you feel the love bubbling in your chest?

The mind is like a receiver, and the thoughts are like frequency. Whatever frequency you are on, that is the channel you are going to pick up and gather information from, and the mind becomes what thoughts it engages in. The body physiology changes accordingly to support the state of mind.

Vitaraaga means 'without raga' - a person who is free from cravings of the world. A person who has no greed, or passion of fulfilment of desires. It is not that desires do not arise – the desires do not inspire feverishness. There is Vairagya. Such a person has a steady mind. One can achieve a steady mind if one thinks of a person who is with a steady mind – it can be your spiritual master, a saint, or any enlightened being.

There is a need to be careful in this practice. A practitioner can become stuck on the person they are contemplating upon. The goal of the practice may be lost. That is why in Indian culture, practitioners are asked to contemplate on their spiritual Master, but reminded that the Master is not a physical entity, but pure consciousness. Otherwise, the practitioner feels separate from the Master, and places the Master at a distance on a pedestal. Since there is a distance, a despair takes root in the mind. Instead of dropping off stagnant thoughts, another illusion is created that become a huge obstacle.

Sri Sri Ravi Shankar was once asked by a devotee that how could he become like him (Sri Sri Ravi Shankar). Sri Sri replied, "You are me. I am you."

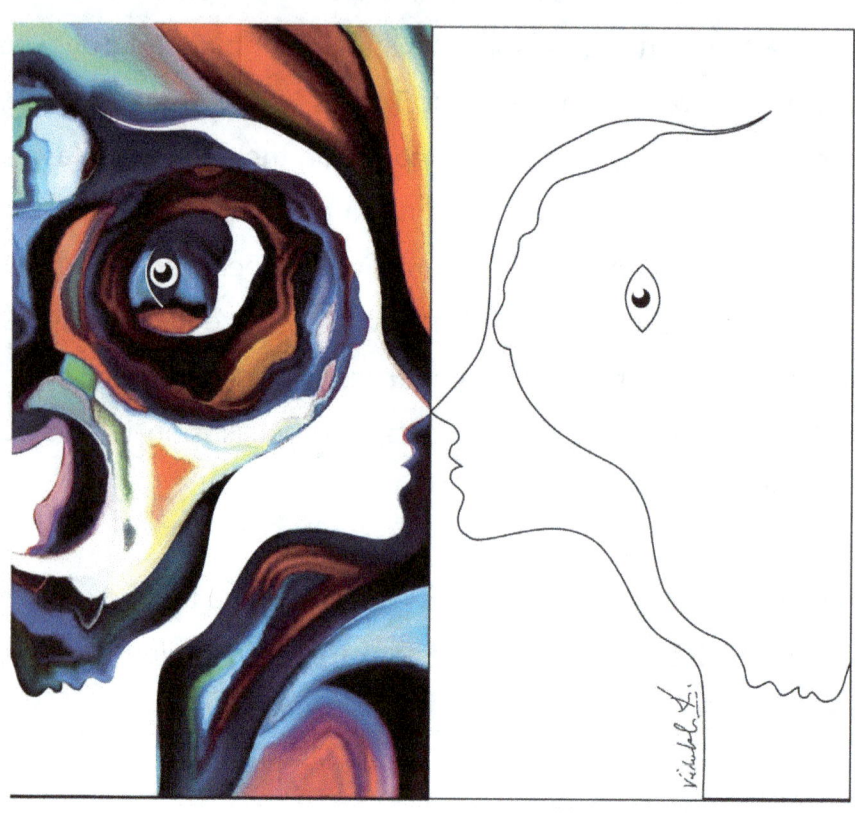

1.38

WIDE ASLEEP

स्वप्ननिद्राज्ञानालम्बनं वा ॥
svapnanidrājñānālambanaṁ vā ॥
(Svapna Nidra Jnana-aalambana vaa)

By witnessing sleep & dreams (the mind can be made steady).

"The moment you know you are sleeping; you are already awake."
- Sri Sri Ravi Shankar

As a human being, we have a great range to experience the variety of the world we live in. This variety is also expressed in our inner worlds – we feel so many different emotions other than happy or sad like anger, jealousy, compassion, curiosity, love, fear, disgust, agony, and so many more which I lack to state not because of my lack of ability to feel but my lack of vocabulary. Words anyway fall short to describe emotions. Yet, I find it quite ironical that we tend to live as if the world is dichotomous.

The two large boxes we have are labelled 'Good' and 'Bad'. We divide them into further smaller boxes of "Right" and "Wrong". Any experience, any thought, any person, any circumstance, and we, consciously or unconsciously, label it as "good" or "bad". Once we have labelled them, they cease to be what they are for us.

Being kind is good. Being jealous is bad. Feeling anger is wrong. Being generous is right. Being productive is good. Resting is unproductive and a waste of time, hence it is bad. God is good, human being is bad. Being rude is bad. Being polite is good. A person is rude once and we label the person as rude. The person is always going to be that "rude person" in our mind instead of just being a person. Even now as you are reading this (and I am writing it) you (and I) have labelled this pattern of labelling as 'bad'. The depth and the possibilities of the concept have been lost. The habit is so intrinsic, our mind cannot stand without it. If we take away the categorization skill of the mind, we suddenly feel our intellects have been handicapped.

This dichotomy does not start from our intellect, but from our instincts. But our instincts cannot be fooled as easily as our intellects. The first dichotomy is the most glaring one which we as a species have been trying to conquer for a long time. Life and Death. We *are either alive or dead.*

What happens when a person dies? They become a nobody – *no body* - no possessions, no family, no friends, and no likes or dislikes. The body is dropped. The senses are lost. No one expects anything of them, and everyone will tell you what a good person they were. It must be a relief to be dead and be free from all the expectations, but for that a good life is necessary first.

We experience this state every day when we sleep. Sleep is quite similar to Death. There are no sensations, no identities, no thoughts. If you had a good day, you would have a good night's sleep as well. It does not matter to your mind whether you are asleep in a castle or a prison cell.

All of us experience the state of wakefulness and sleep and dreams. But there is another state that is beyond these. There is an interface where we are neither asleep, nor awake. The quality of being awake is described as being in activity and motion. The senses are active – we see, we hear, we smell, and we taste. Our individuality and ego are expressed. The brain analyses the information from the senses, and we act accordingly. The quality of sleep is the lack of sensations. We lose our sense of self.

But in the interface, we are awake, but there are no thoughts (until we want) but a pervading awareness. The sense of self exists, but it encompasses not only the body and mind, but all the space around us. The eyes see, but get to make a choice if we want to process what we see. We are able to listen, see, feel and process without any veil of our desires and emotions. There is power. There is control. There is connection - our existence expands from a small body to Nature itself.

Being aware in sleep is one of the toughest sadhanas. Sadhguru of Isha Foundation also mentions this sadhana in his books and talks. Bhagavan Ramana Maharishi has also talked about the state in which one becomes aware of the sleeping state. You can try it for yourself. When you lie down to sleep tonight, simply try to observe your mind slipping into the sleeping state. It is extremely hard, and needs a lot of regular practice of being continuously aware of the activity of the mind beforehand to witness sleep, but you can still give it a try. I have experienced it once during my teacher training program. I was doing rigorous sadhana every day, and was in the grace of the Master. Watching myself sleep was one of the strangest experiences of my life, and when I woke up, I was not sure if I had really slept that night or not. It took me some time to realize that I had actually been able to witness the vrittis of sleep for the entire night.

The Masters like Sadhguru and Ramana Maharishi have given an easier way to observe this state. Instead of observing the state while going into sleep, observe it when coming out of sleep. There are a few seconds when we are waking up from sleep that we can be aware. At the moment, we are neither asleep, nor awake; we are in a transcendental state. If we learn to observe this state, and slowly hold the awareness even while we are awake, the mind can go into Samadhi.

In Bhagavad Gita, Lord Krishna says that the Yogi is asleep when the ordinary people are awake, and awake when the ordinary people are asleep. Adi Shankarcharaya explains what the Lord is saying - The enlightened being understands that all he is seeing is a dream, and not true. They are asleep to its effects, and are not swayed, as one is not swayed by a dream, not matter how extraordinary it might have been. Ordinary people, in their ignorance, believe this dream to be true and keep on struggling and resisting. Take a minute and look back. Is not your life like a dream? Eating, sleeping, working, talking, crying, laughing...it is all transient. The "awake" truth is flowing, changing with time – if the awareness does not flow with it, are we experiencing truth?

But there is something in us that is real and has not changed at all, and the only few moments in our life that have really stayed with us are those in which we experienced the vastness of our existence, our unchanging core that is pure.

Become aware of sleep, see that it is all a dream. Remember the transience of all. In the words of John Green "We are small, and so frail, so gloriously and terrifyingly temporary."

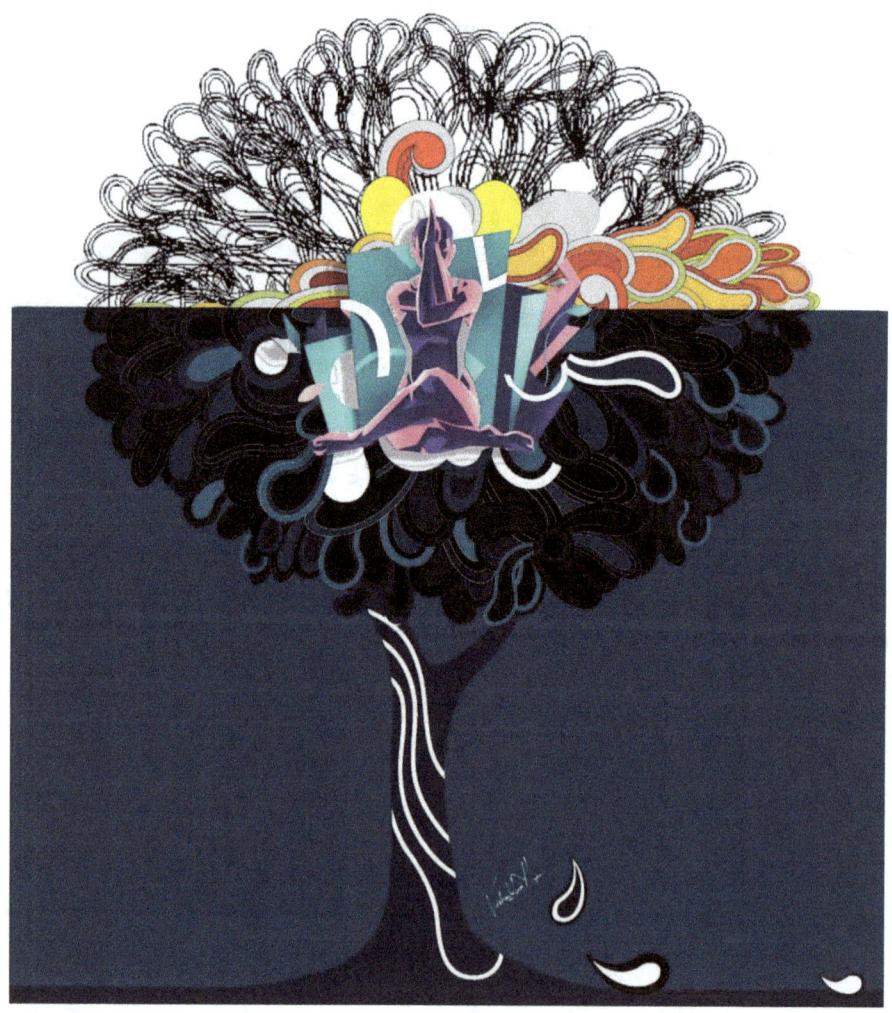

1.39

AS YOU LIKE IT

यथाभिमतध्यानाद्वा ॥
Yathābhimatadhyānādvā ॥
(yathaa abhimat Dhyaanaad vaa)

By meditating on what one likes
(the mind can be made steady).

"Anything you accept fully will get you there."
- Eckhart Tolle

Hisako Koyama was born while World War I was raging. Born at a time when and in a community where young girls were not pushed to have professional careers, she was fortunate to have a family which valued education. She loved watching the sky, and her father encouraged her enthusiasm by getting her a refractive telescope.

During the second World War, blackouts regularly hit the city of Tokyo to prepare and deal with airstrikes. Sirens would have blared; lights would be extinguished. People must have run for shelter clutching at their hearts and loved ones. Yet, for this young girl, it was an opportunity to gaze at the twinkling little lights in the night sky, which looked even better above the blacked-out city. While big men with great power and greater egos fought and sneaked to steal little but dirt, a young girl would sneak out and steal the stars.

This was the beginning of a love affair between a young girl and our own star, the Sun. Koyama went on to spend her entire life inspecting the sun and sketching it. Her meticulous observations and sunspot drawings went on to shape the modern field of space weather, and is the foundation of solar study which is critical in building all kinds of satellites and space probes.

She inspected the sun and hand-drew each blemish and sun spot every-day for than 40 years – more than 15000 days, and unimaginable number of hours.

The story of Hisako Koyama grounds me on both the good and the bad days. On the days when I feel anxiety overpowering me, I am reminded and assured of the resilience we are capable of. On the days my mind bloats with ego, I am reminded of how a young girl accomplished more during war than most of manage in times of peace.

But more than anything, there is a sense of kinship when I look up at the stars - I am reminded how the human species have been enraptured by the night sky across space and time. I am reminded our capability to love not just one another, but the sun, moon, and stars. Koyama was not a genius. She was ordinary – and her extraordinary trait was she did not try to become extraordinary. She liked doing something and she did it day after day, every day. She might not have even known what would be the use of her extensive study. But she achieved that only few of us ever aspire for, and ever fewer ever achieve – single-minded dispassion. I can only imagine the tranquility of her presence, the softness of her mind, and the gentleness of her voice.

All these techniques, all these tricks to fool the mind are not necessary. Simply find one thing that we like and focusing our mind on it like a laser, and doing it incessantly – this is the key. It is no big secret. It is simple.

Do not worry about gazing at a light, or listening to a flute, or remembering an enlightened being. Do not put effort in holding your breath. The only thing which is not going to help, is to keep on jumping from one sadhana to another because someone told you about the lights they saw, or the sounds the heard in meditation, or how sharp they had become by doing a sadhana. Let us choose one thing to dedicate ourselves to as we live. Let us practice it with honor and reverence, day in and day out. Let our practice become the goal. Let everything come to us.

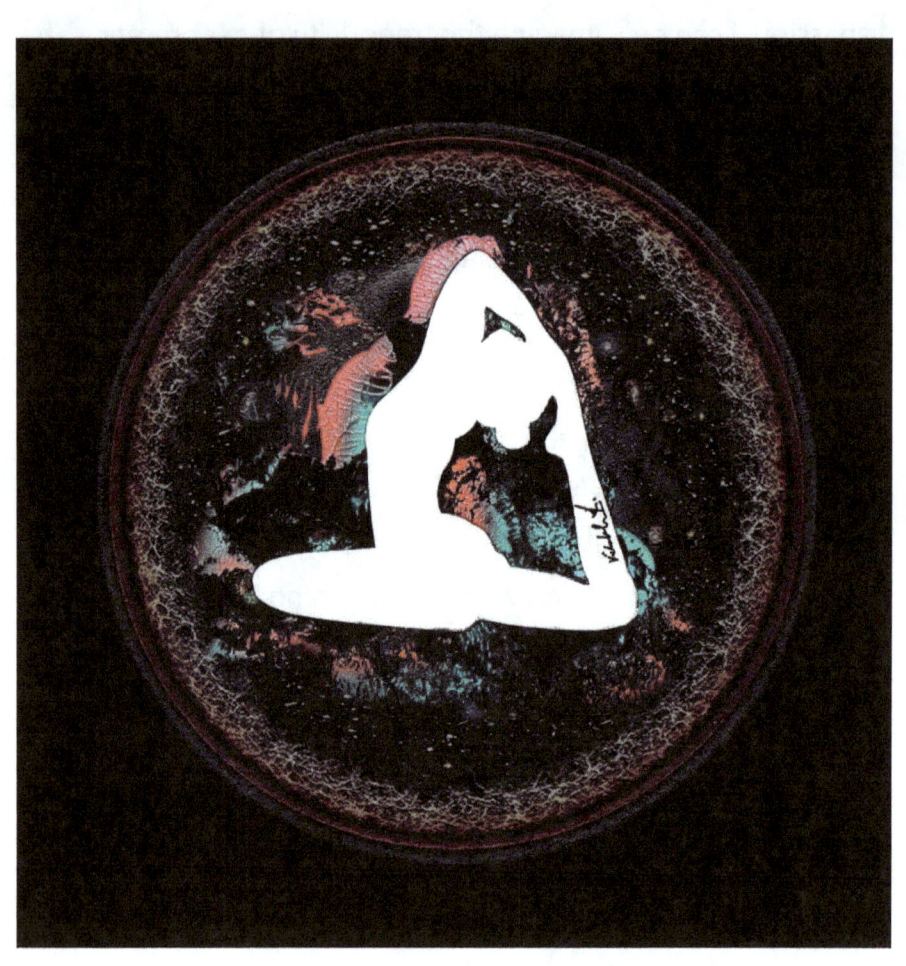

1.40

WORLD IN THE PALM OF MY HAND

परमाणुपरममहत्त्वान्तोऽस्य वशीकारः ॥
paramāṇuparamamahattvānto'sya vaśīkāraḥ ॥
(Paramaanu parama Mahattva anta asya Vashikaara)

The practitioner gains control over the smallest as well as the infinitely large.

"When I look inside and see that I am Nothing, that is Wisdom. When I look outside and see that I'm everything, that is Love. And between these two, my Life turns."
- Nisargadatta Maharaj

The story of Sri Krishna and Sudama is well known in India. Childhood friends who studied together, Sri Krishna became the King of Dwarka, and Sudama lived a Brahmin's life. At that time, it was a rule to live on alms for a Brahmin, and it was considered a privilege to give alms to a Brahmin. But Sudama was the poorest of the poor. Encouraged by his wife to ask Sri Krishna for help, Sudama reluctantly reaches Dwarka. A frail man, skin barely hanging to his bones and bloody feet, with dirt in every pore of his skin and a thin cloth to cover his trembling body, stood at the gates of Dwarka. The guards refused to believe that this was a friend of their King. Yet, brahmins were not to be turned away in Krishna's Dwarka. Krishna was informed. Krishna dropped everything and he ran. Krishna sat Sudama on his throne and washed his feet – the King became the servant of the poorest, but he was not a King when he welcomed and hosted Sudama...he was a friend, hosting an old friend who was weary from travel as well as life. There was no status, no ego, no pride. On receiving such respect and honor, and being treated like an equal, Sudama could not being himself to ask Krishna for any help.

When Sudama returned home, he found a well-built house instead of his dilapidated hut. His children were well-fed and well-clothed. This was the work of a King – how could a kingdom prosper if a pious man of honor, integrity, and knowledge could not support his family and they were all dying of hunger? Why would then anyone go in pursuit of knowledge? Why would anyone be proud of integrity? Why would anyone have faith in a King? It would simply destroy the kingdom for people would give up these qualities. Even as a King, Sri Krishna was a dasa.

A great person understands the fragility of his own existence. In his own self, he is a nobody. He does not take himself too seriously. In his outer self, he is aware of how life is interconnected – each and everything affects each and everything. Nothing is outside Life. John Green put it beautifully in The Anthropocene Reviewed, "All life is dependent on other life, and the closer we consider what constitutes living, the harder life becomes to define." In this sense, he is everybody and everything. He cannot be indifferent. Yet his internal state makes sure is also never feverish or afraid. There is control over the smallest and the largest of issues. There is balance.

But from chaos comes order. Sleep comes to those who are awake during the day. Effortlessness blossoms in those who cross the limit of effort. Balance comes to those who have fallen innumerable times and yet continue forward without blaming and complaining. So, it is not an easy path. It is not easy to simply be – to be receptive of each second and experience eternity in it. This is the result of a steady mind, one which has been decluttered and steadied, should one be brave enough to aim for it.

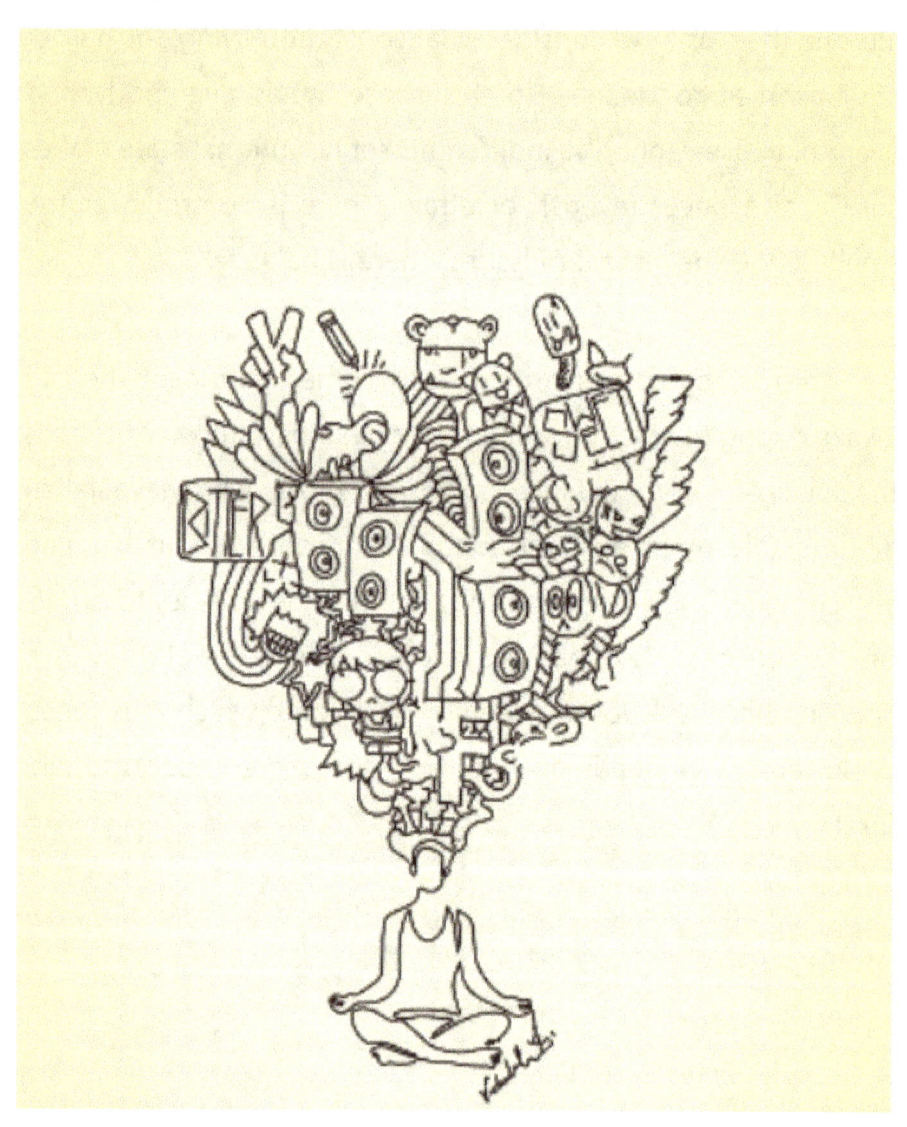

1.41

ETERNAL SUNSHINE OF THE SPOTLESS MIND

क्षीणवृत्तेरभिजातस्येव मणेर्ग्रहीतृग्रहणग्राह्येषु तत्स्थतदञ्जनतासमापत्तिः ॥
kṣīṇavṛtterabhijātasyeva maṇergrahītṛgrahaṇagrāhyeṣu tatsthatadañjanatāsamāpattiḥ ॥
(Kshina vrtte, Abhijaatasya iva mane, Grahitr-Grahana-Graahyeshu, Tatstha Tatanjanataa Samaapatti)

When the mind becomes free of its modulations, it becomes like a pure reflecting crystal, and plays the role of the Seer, Seeing, and Seen; effortlessly in the moment.

"The mind is like a photographic plate. It clicks pictures of the events, but the events are not there."
- Sri Sri Ravi Shankar

We sat together in the amphitheatre, our legs touching. The sky was a brilliant blue above us. The air smelt of the earth after rain, and a light breeze caressed our skin. I sensed a stillness deep within me, and it oozed out to my senses, such that everything I perceived seemed to deepen the calm.

'It was the best experience of my life. I had never known such peace and bliss.' My voice was barely a whisper.

'Hmm...' – she nodded – 'I hope you get to experience that again.'

The silence within me broke. I realised that, no matter how hard I tried, I could not communicate my experience with anyone. A laugh escaped deep from my chest. 'No', I said. 'The moment was complete. The experience was fulfilling. I have no desire or need to experience that again.'

The new pandemic of the modern world (besides Covid) is the overwhelming fixation on future. All kinds of people, because of the easy reach to the masses, suddenly have become convinced that what they know and the way they live their life is the only way to live. This conviction brings a kind of self-belief and power over one's presence and words that can easily influence those who have self-doubt. Today, if I open social media, everyone is a "gyaani" – a wise one. Everyone is giving out advice – how to think, how to act, what opinion to have (and not to have), and how to have a good *future*. People of all ages including children and teens are being told that food, sleep and rest is for losers. Celebration is a waste of time. The only way to live today is to *hustle* until you cannot keep your eyes open and then hustle some more. If you are not outworking the other person, you are not working enough. Even right now, if you think about it, I am writing to give you some knowledge as if I know some secret. I, fortunately, do not labor under the delusion that my way of life is the only productive way of life, or that I know something that others are incapable of knowing. It is quite liberating to be ordinary. I believe that every life has its own shape and path, and every person must find their own truth. No one can give it to you.

J. Krishnamurti puts it succinctly:
"Truth cannot be accumulated."

The obsession with making the future better has a simple implication – the present moment is an obstacle to be dealt with. We will be happy tomorrow because tomorrow will be better than today – today, we must struggle. But, tomorrow never comes. Only our imagination is thriving in the present, and our imagination is scared, because everyone keeps telling us that if we do not have a life they have, if we do not live by *their* morals, if we do not make *them* proud, then we have failed at life. It breeds self-doubt, and one day, we are not sure if we should listen to ourselves anymore. It feels easier to let someone else tell us what life means and how to live it. Suddenly, we find ourselves running around to do something someone else told us to do, to build a life someone else told us we would be happy to have using the tools we do not know if are compatible for us. A few days later, someone else will come along and tell you something different, and your mind will take off like a bullet in the other direction. What a joke! No wonder we are exhausted. No wonder the world seems so heavy and scary.

Where is life? Neither the past exists, nor the future – these exist in our memory and imagination respectively. Memory is seldom accurate, and our imagination has already been hijacked along with half of our intellect. We are half dead, not because we do not have, but because we have been *told* that what we have is the not the right thing to have, and what we will have tomorrow will be better and it is not right to be happy and content now. We are told that we cannot think for ourselves, that we are unintelligent, unwise, and uncomprehending in the face of the truth of life which only *they* seem to know. Life is passing like a dream, foggy and always just out of grasp.

The mind does not like noise. It likes space. It literally becomes aware of life when it is not occupied with anything in particular – neuroimaging shows that areas of brain associated with the sense of self are not active in people who are always stressed. When the mind is steadied, it becomes soft and receptive. A passive awareness develops that flows with the time – keeping with the present. The present, instead of a foe to be wrestled, becomes a friend to share silence with. The nature of being human starts to express, and since it is *nature*, it is natural. One discovers oneself – our needs, our inclinations, our strength, and our weakness. It is now impossible not to take decisions that yield what we desire to achieve. Acceptance develops. Compassion flows. Then, life is content, and yet every action is fulfilling.

The mind becomes pure like a reflecting crystal, pure and untainted by anything it comes in contact with. Every moment is experienced in its entirety, in its endless depth, and when it passes, the mind does not hold on to the desire of the joy, or the fear of pain in the moment. Such a person goes beyond space and time, for each moment becomes eternal and infinite – the present never runs out. Such a mind is free – and such a mind has achieved Yoga.

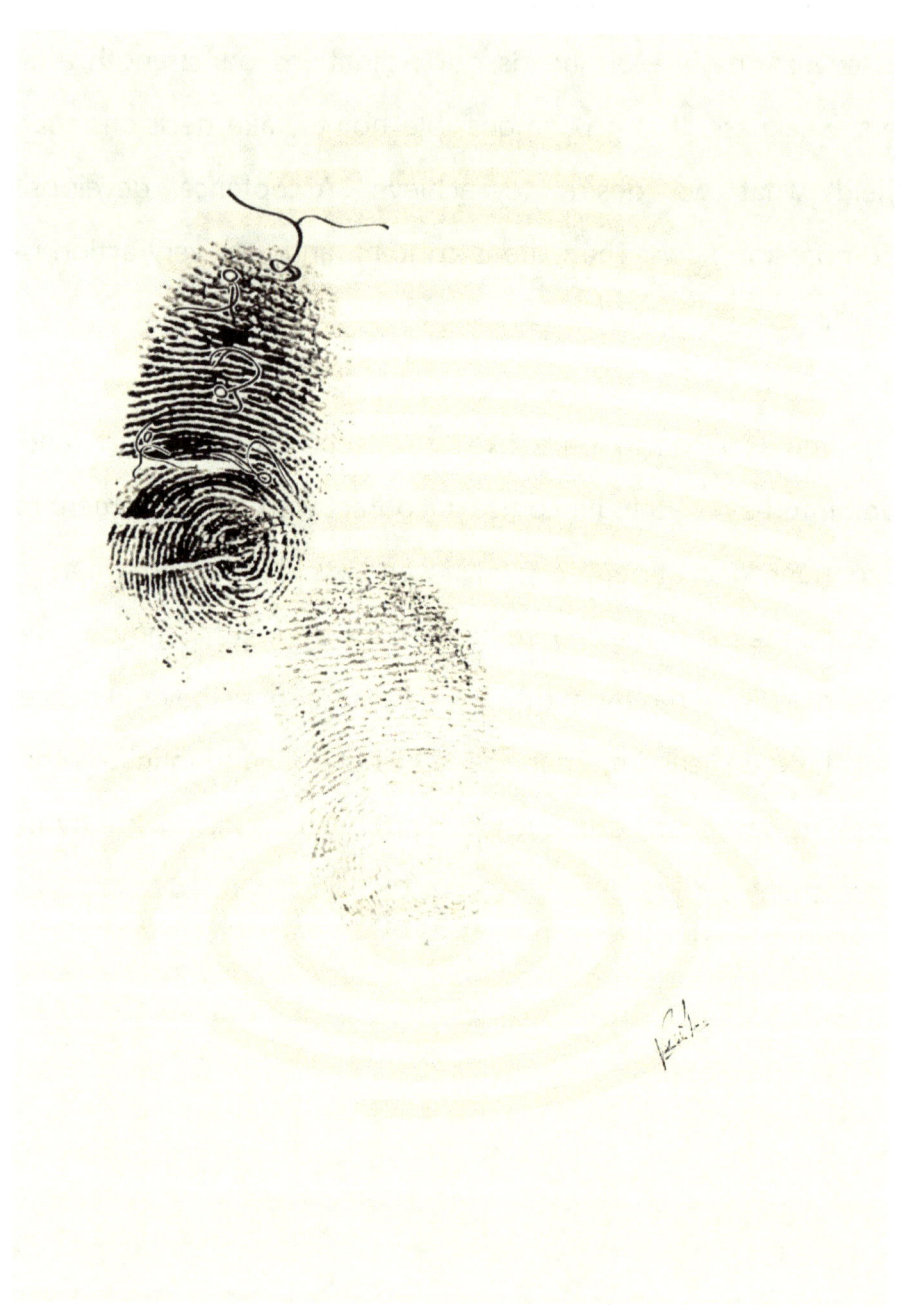

1.42

WHAT'S IN A NAME?

तत्र शब्दार्थज्ञानविकल्पैः संकीर्णा सवितर्का समापत्तिः ॥
tatra śabdārthajñānavikalpaiḥ saṁkīrṇā savitarkā samāpattiḥ ॥
(tatra Shabda, Artha, Jnaana, vikalpai sankeernaa Savitarkaa Samaapatti)

The samadhi state in which the word, its meaning, and its deeper knowledge; alternate in the mind, is known as Savitarka Samapatti.

"Mind is Space, Thinking is Time."
- Ashwini Aggarwal, Conversations with Space

Humans took over the Earth primarily due to three reasons: extensive imagination, ability to communicate the imagination, and ability to get a large number to believe in that imagination and turn a lot of it into reality.

Paper money works because everyone believes the paper means something; if one day, everyone decided that the printed dollar is trash, it will literally become trash. Thousands of people work for a company – an imaginary, non-living entity that exists only as a name on paper (even people exist on paper now-a-days: there was a case in India in which a man went to court for more than a decade to prove he is alive because some official document said he was dead) – and profess loyalty for it and its vision and mission. The imaginative identity goes as far as to have a name, its own money, land, and other assets. Talk about "talking about reality."

The act of communicating the imagination and ideas requires a language. Conversely, for a thought to arise, a language is needed to think.

Language is a collection of symbols with a form, and an object. Spoken languages, have a third element that is sound. When you read the word CHAIR, what happens? Try reading the word a few times slowly and observe how the three dimensions of the symbol– form, sound, and object – are revealed. If you sit with the word a little longer, your mind will start generating characteristics of the object like weight, height, and color.

Therefore, for a thought to arise, a language is critical. Research shows people with a greater vocabulary, or those who are multilingual, have a clearer and more refined internal dialogue than others, and even happen to have a better hold on their emotional state.

When you read the word CHAIR, you are reciting a sound in your head which you learned in primary school – "cheair".

That is what reading the word means – make the combination of sounds che-air for the combination of symbols c-h-a-i-r. The form of the symbol is the Roman Alphabet and the name is che-air. We also learnt that the object of the symbol is a seat generally with 4 legs and a back rest. Now, we are unable to look at this word without making the sound in our head, and generating the picture of the object on the mental screen. It is so because we have become conditioned.

Let us approach this from another direction. Look at the chair for a few seconds and do not think of anything else. Simply stare at the chair as if you have a crush on it. Well, what happened? If you stare at the chair without any intention, your mind might have given you the name of the object without you asking for it, but after some time, all that you saw was the object. The name vanished. The object does not contain the name, but, as we experimented earlier, the name has the object. Any object has a name, form, and its attributes (knowledge). When one starts to sit for meditation, we get a lot of thoughts. In meditation, we do not suppress the thoughts, we observe them and let them flow. In Savitarka Samadhi, the name of the object, the form of the object, and the sound are not separate. These attributes of the object keep on intermingling. The intellect is at play, but the contemplation on the single object is effortless.

There is no other object in the mind, but the name, form and knowledge of the object are yet to be separated. In this Samadhi, a lot of ideas may be generated about the object which may not have been generated before. Many problems resolve here on their own.

S. Ramanujan, one of the greatest mathematicians, once said that he saw solutions to mathematical problems in his sleep. He was completely and wholly engrossed in mathematical research and his intellect produced results even passively.

This form of Samadhi is the first step to Samadhi and need the mind to be emptied of distractions. Only then the object assimilates with the mind fully, and greater knowledge of the object is revealed to the intellect of the mind.

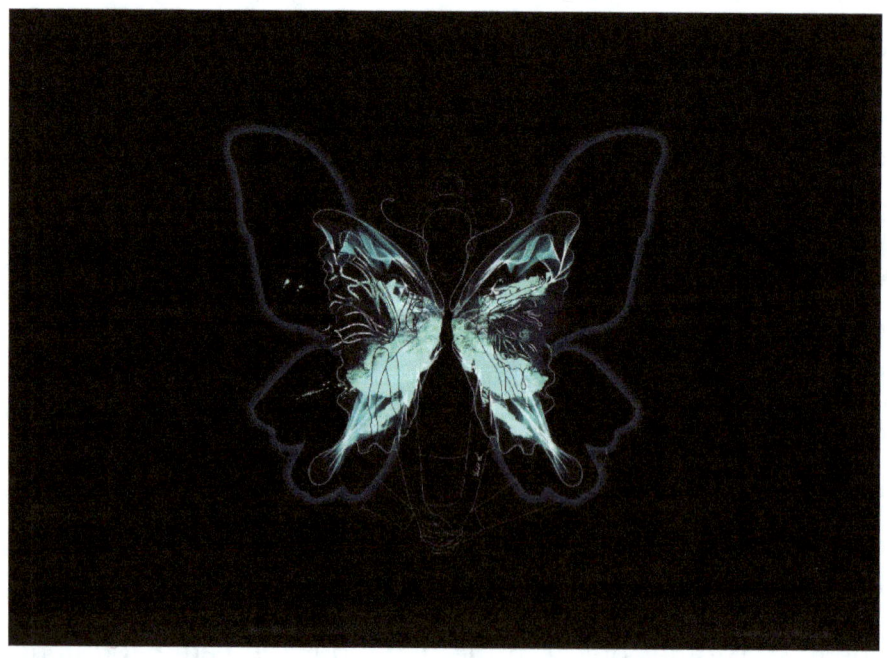

1.43

EMPTINESS

स्मृतिपरिशुद्धौ स्वरूपशून्येवार्थमात्रनिर्भासा निर्वितर्का ॥
smṛtipariśuddhau svarūpaśūnyevārthamātranirbhāsā nirvitarkā ॥
(Smriti-parishudhau, Svaroopa-shoonya iva, Artha-maatra nirbhaasaa Nirvitarkaa)

When the memory is purified, the mind becomes devoid of its self-awareness, and only the object remains illuminated; this is Nirvitarka.

"Know that any situation, any person, can change at any time."
- Gurudev Sri Sri Ravi Shankar

For a large part, our impressions in the memory are the basis of our identity. We identify ourselves as a gender, as a relation, as a position, as a title, etc. and as such do we identify others. Then the impressions of the past events superimpose on our perception of our present events, causing us to err in our perception and generating further impressions. The memory becomes clouded, and becomes a jumble of associations, and the awareness of the self is buried under fragmented perceptions. Most of us have an inherent trust on our memory, but in truth it has poor reliability. Research and experiments have shown that memory can be easily manipulated, so much so that, an innocent person can be convinced to confess to a crime with all the details of place, time and person even if they had never ever been to that place in their lives. What is to tell us that our memories regarding other events are truly accurate?

A clean/pure memory does not mean that there is no record of the events that have passed. Such a person, as can be imagined, would not be able to navigate any dimension of life, and would suffer from great trauma. A purified memory means where the associations have been unlearned, and the awareness is always fresh and error free. A purified memory is one which does not interfere until voluntary accessed.

In Savitarka samadhi, the memory is not purified. The learned knowledge about the object keeps on mingling with the name and form of the object. Learned ideas provide input about the object. The intellect continues to work. The name, the form, and the knowledge of the object are not yet distinct. The thoughts are arising, scenes from the memory are replayed, but the consciousness gains the ability to sit back and just observe, instead of going on a ride itself. The mind and the object/thought are two separate entities and the awareness of the distinction between the two components exists. The mind continues to try and work out the object, fetching reason and past data from the memory. It so happens that after a while, the awareness of observing the thoughts also disappears. The memory disappears. All that exists is the present. The thoughts continue to arise and run, but the consciousness goes into a deep rest, where it is not aware. The observer on the bank watching the river run by realises that it is the same water, going through endless cycles. It lies down, and stares at the great, pure blue sky. Slowly the eyes close, and Nothing remains. It becomes Space. There is emptiness.

In this state of Nirvitarka Samadhi, the memory is purified. The logical faculties go to rest – you stop analysing and just experience what is without super imposing any association from your memory. We cannot remember what garbage, or which memory or impression has been removed from the mind, for it does not exist in the consciousness anymore. The mind starts to become burden free, soft, and light.

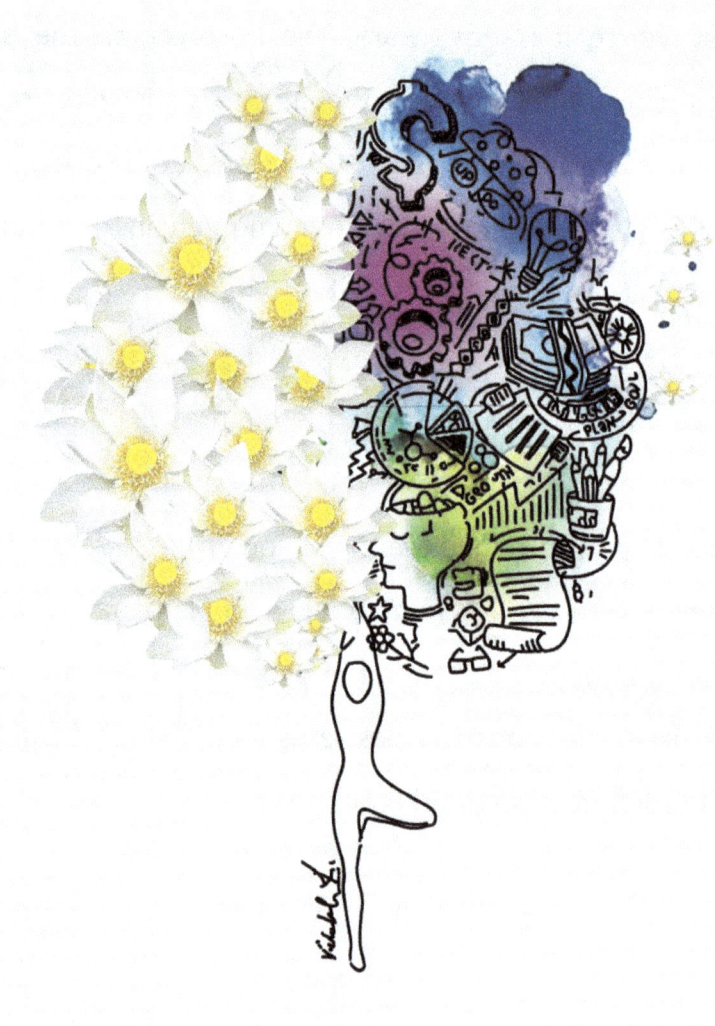

1.44

CHEWING GUM

एतयैव सविचारा निर्विचारा च सूक्ष्मविषया व्याख्याता ॥
etayaiva savicārā nirvicārā ca sūkṣmaviṣayā vyākhyātā ॥
(etayaiva Savichara Nirvichara ca suksham-vishayaa vyaakhyaataa)

Similarly, are explained Savichara and Nirvichara Samadhi, which are the subtler states of consciousness.

"Here Vichara means Experiences – Anubhuti."
- Gurudev Sri Sri Ravi Shankar

Subtler than the memory are our experiences. Experiences are a form of memory too; they are what our personality has become, and our attitude towards different aspects of life; experiences are reflected in our likes and dislikes, our patterns that we identify with so closely that we are unable to recognise them. Experiences are stored deep in our consciousness, beyond intellect, and many times, beyond recall as well. Experiences are what form our identity.

In Savichara Samadhi, the experiences exist and start to surface. Also, there is the experience of the Samadhi itself. Once the experiences surface and can be witnessed, they become separate from our being. There is an opportunity to discover and realise that the experiences are not what we are, but what we have accumulated. The experiences are simply deep impressions in our memory.

This sense of being distinct from we have experienced begs the question – Who am I? I am not the body, not the mind, not the memory and not the experiences. All these are what we have accumulated. What did we come with then? When one starts to view oneself separate from the impression of events that we have stored as experiences, there sprouts an inquiry of our true nature of being.

From here, one dives into Nirvichara Samadhi – a state in which the practitioner does not witness any impressions of the experiences. There is no experience of the Samadhi, and hence, the practitioner is simply being. When there are no experiences present in the accessed consciousness, there is no sense of time and space as well, for there is no past or future, there is no accumulated identity of body, mind, or memory, and one loses contact with the boundary of the physical dimension we hold ourselves in. It must be understood that in Nirvichara Samadhi, it is not that the impressions have been deleted. It is just that the consciousness dips a little deeper where the impressions do not exist. Samadhi is a spectrum of the consciousness, and it is fluid state – one can move from one state to another (even multiple times) in a single sitting.

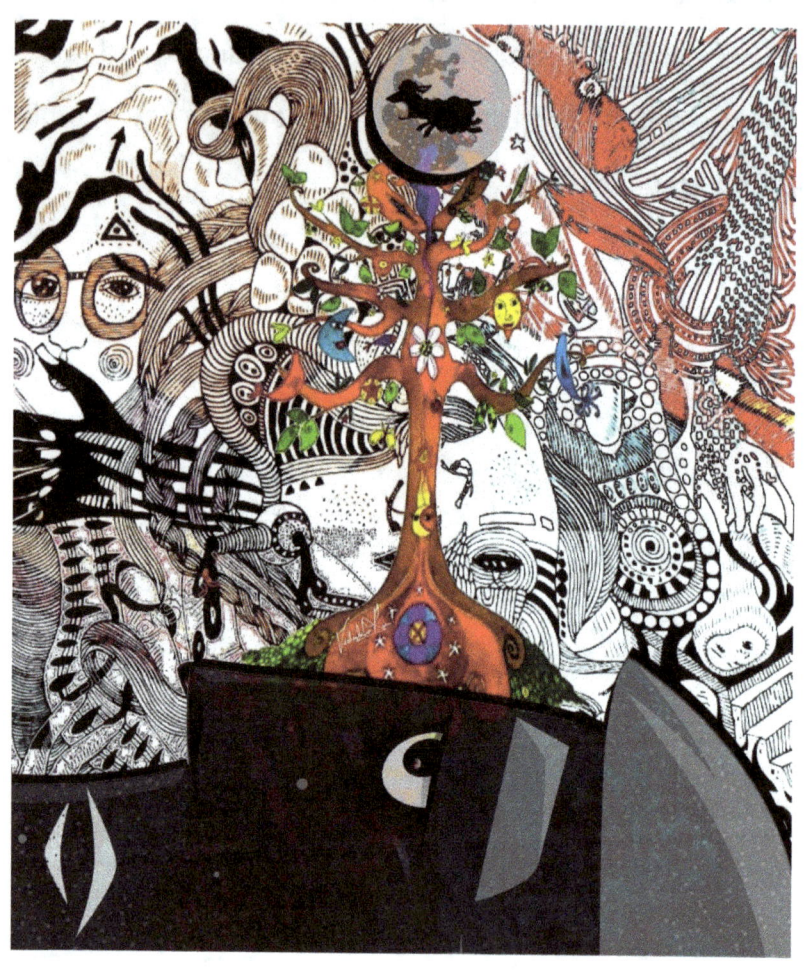

1.45

BRUCE ALMIGHTY

सूक्ष्मविषयत्वं चालिङ्गपर्यवसानम् ॥
sūkṣmaviṣayatvaṁ cāliṅgaparyavasānam ॥
(Suksham vishayatvam ca aaling pari-avsaanam)

Of the subtle objects, the conclusion is the Unmanifest.

"And forget not that the earth delights to feel your bare feet and the winds long to play with your hair."
-Khalil Gibran

The world we are sensitized to and perceive is that which is obvious and evident. We are not aware of the taste of the wind, or the mood of the clouds. We do not feel the flight of the eagle in our muscles, nor the trees pushing to the skies. We cannot sense the energies flowing within us, much less than the energies working in the earth, the oceans, the sun, moon, and the stars.

There is a subtle world at play, which is many times more potent and sensitive, affected by every thought, intention, and desire, not just of human beings (we like to believe we are special, but we are not *that* special), but of every rock, puddle, tree, animal, and blade of grass. Our senses are not able to perceive the depth and payers of the universe because we are stuck in our 8'x8' cubicles with our laptops and mobile phones. We have forgotten to sit with the trees, and if and when we see them, we forget they see us too. We do not walk barefoot on the earth anymore, and if and when we do, we fail to realize that the earth yearns for our touch too. The wind longs to move through our bones, and the rain comes down because that is the only way for the heavens to descend and feel the warmth of our skin. We, as a species, have forgotten that everything that we sense, everything that we perceive, is based on the principle of reciprocity – the sensible is also sensing. Every moment is a transaction where the senses and sensible nourish each other.

In the Samkhya Philosophy, Purusha and Prakriti are the two aspects of the universe. Purusha is Shiva – the Supreme Consciousness, beyond space and time, that which is without any form, quality, or nature. Prakriti is Shakti – the manifest principle of Shiva, which assumes form. Prakriti is the cause of all that is manifest, from subtlest to the most gross. Rising from Prakriti to Purusha, that is union of the manifest with the causal unmanifest is the true union which we call Yoga.

In the subtler states of Samadhi, when our consciousness is not stuck in our memories, and the impressions of the experiences have been removed; we are not reacting to the world with pre-set conditioner behaviors and ideas, there is no desire to achieve anything, when we are part of the rhythm of the earth, sun and the stars, there is a harmony with the existence. There is an expansion of the consciousness beyond the good and bad, right and wrong, this and that. Then, the subtle realm of the universe is also revealed.

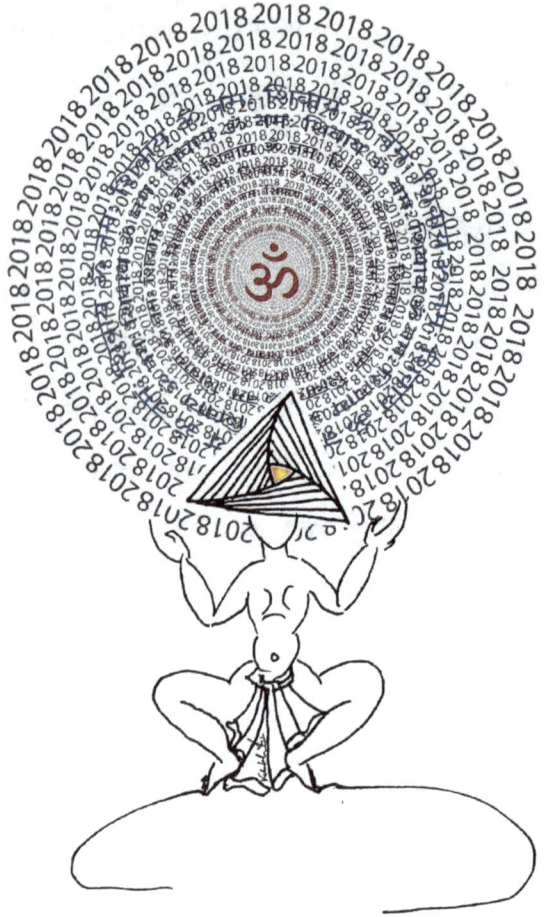

1.47

I AM THAT

निर्विचारवैशारद्येऽध्यात्मप्रसादः ॥

nirvicāravaiśāradye'dhyātmaprasādaḥ ॥

(Nirvichara vaishaaradye Adhyatama Prasada)

Proficiency in Nirvichara bestows divine grace.

As one practices Nirvichara Samadhi regularly, one is again and again going beyond the distinction between the experience and experiencer. There are no two – the merge happens. It must be noted that Patanjali makes sure to mention that it must be practiced regularly. It is not a one-time touch-and-go phenomenon. Because the seed of impressions still exists, the person will have to go through situations and circumstances, that can cause many more impressions – causing the person to make new associations, and identify again with desires, fear, and attachments, keeping the person bound in the cycle.

Only divine grace can work on the seed of latent impressions. This grace is obtained when one masters Nirvichara Samadhi.

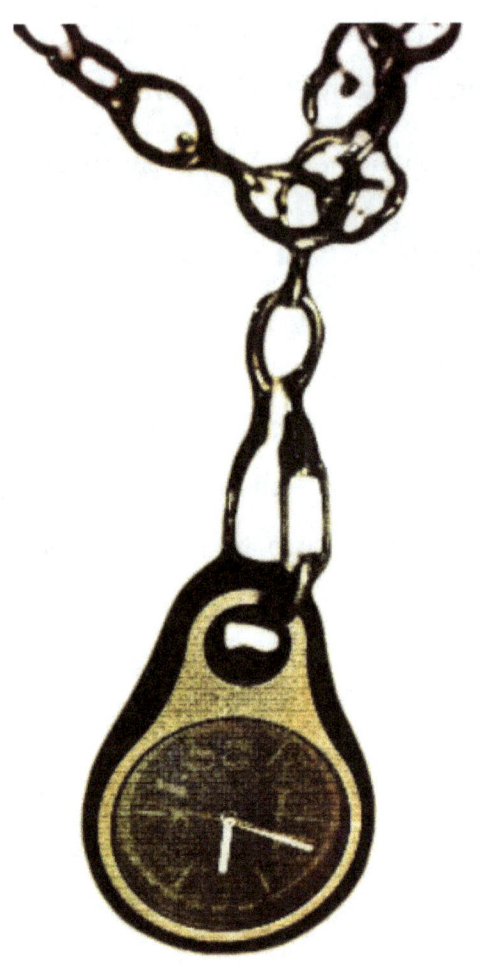

1.48

THE ABSOLUTE

ऋतम्भरा तत्र प्रज्ञा ॥

ṛtambharā tatra prajñā ॥

(Rtambhraa tatra Pragyaa)

Awareness holds nothing but the Truth.

The universe is ever changing. A billion galaxies, and a trillion, trillion stars, being born and dying every day. There is motion and activity. Oe affects the whole and the whole affects the one. A person who has is practicing Nirvichara Samadhi is free of impressions. He gains insight into the interconnectedness of events, and the knowledge that dawns is one of truth and wisdom that is infallible.

Now that which is changing is not absolute. It is Satyam – it is true at that moment, but not outside time. Ṛtam is the absolute truth that is eternal, without a beginning or an end. This is the cause of everything and itself without cause. The consciousness accesses the causal realm, which is beyond the subtle realm as well, and realizes the absolute Truth.

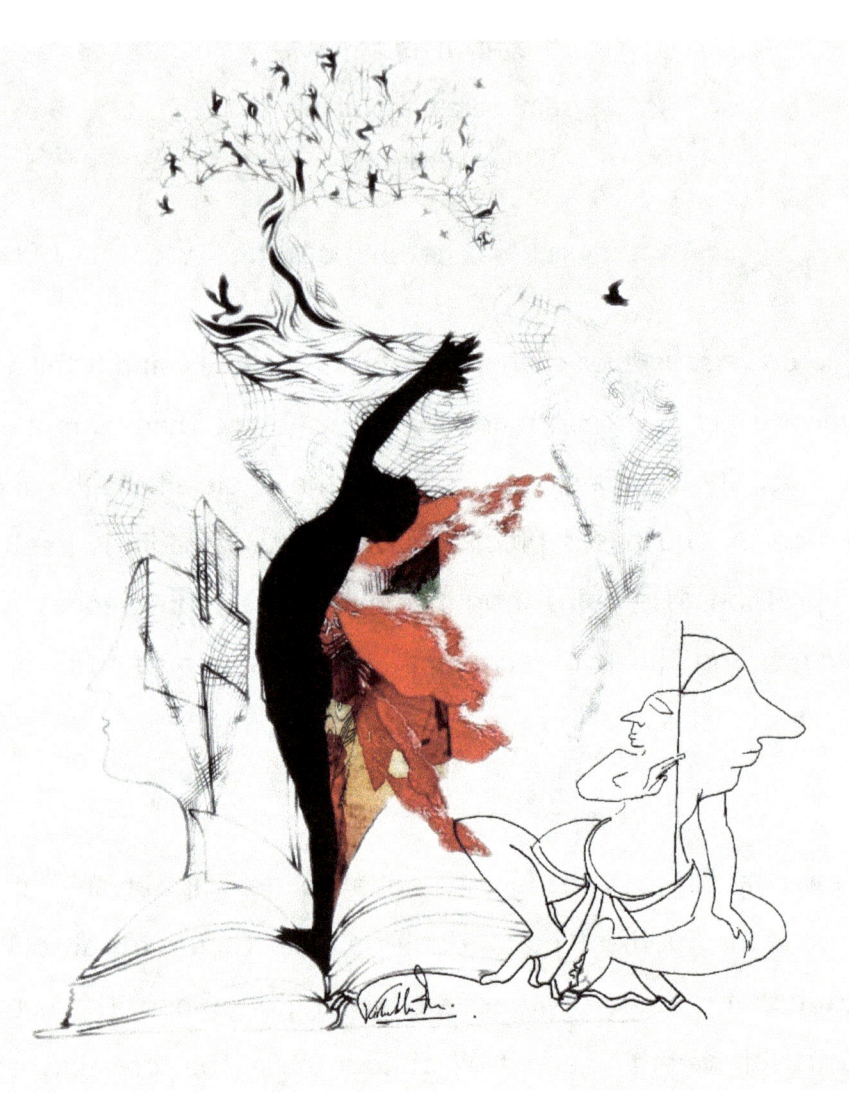

1.49

BREAKING DAWN

श्रुतानुमानप्रज्ञाभ्यामन्यविषया विशेषार्थत्वात् ॥
śrutānumānaprajñābhyāmanyaviṣayā viśeṣārthatvāt ॥
(Shruta Anumana Pragyabhyam, anya vishayaa vishesha arthatvaat)

The knowledge thus obtained is higher than that obtained from inference or hearing.

In Hindu Philosophy, there are two types of knowledge – Shruti and Smriti.

Smriti is that which has been memories; it is that which has been obtained through the senses – by reading in a book, or hearing from a teacher, or from the subtler senses. And it has been rationalized by the intellect. Shruti is knowledge that has been revealed. It is revealed in the state of Samadhi when the awareness has connected to the cosmic consciousness, to the absolute truth. Vedas, Upanishads, and many other Shastras are Shruti Knowledge – they were revealed in the deepest states of Samadhi. Hence, they are not said to be authored, but only revealed.

The truth that is brought into awareness from this Samadhi is flawless; there is no mistake about it. It is different from that which has been learnt from a teacher, or a book, or which has been obtained through inference. It is complete. Such knowledge satisfies the perpetual thirst for knowledge that is the trademark of a human being.

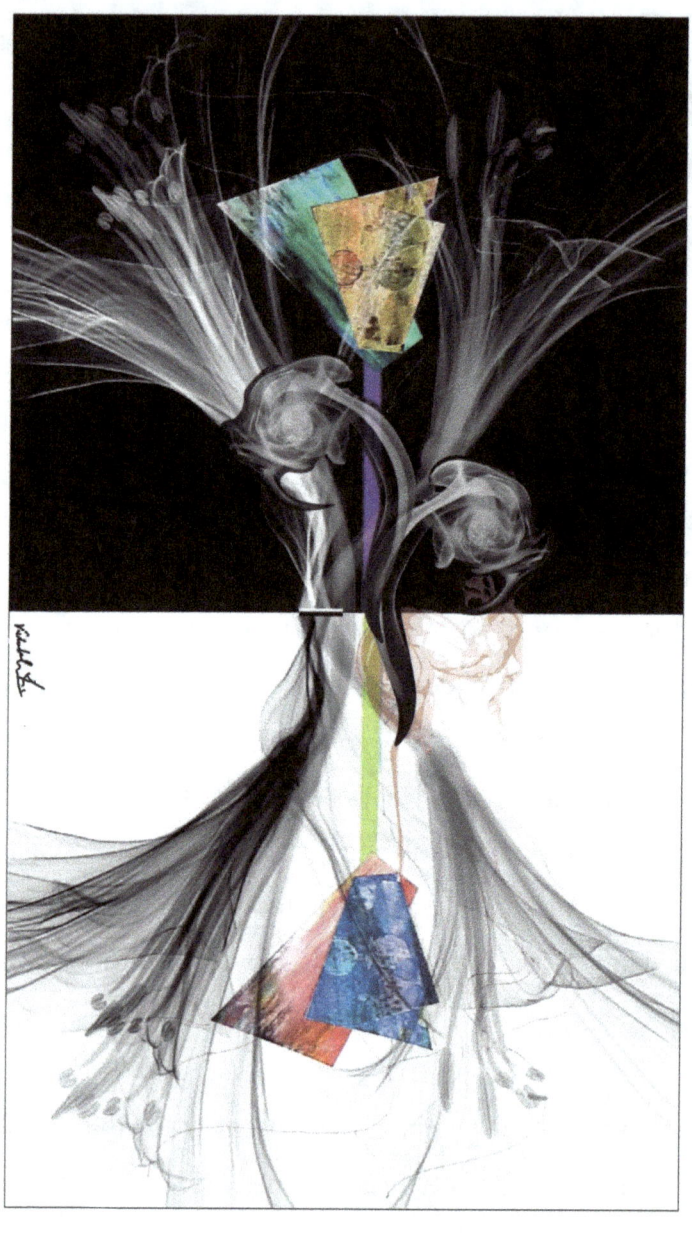

1.50

THE SEED OF CREATION

तज्जः संस्कारोऽन्यसंस्कारप्रतिबन्धी ॥
tajjaḥ saṁskāro'nyasaṁskārapratibandhī ॥
(tatjah Samskara Anya-samskara Pratibandhi)

Impressions born of this Knowledge override the previous impressions.

The knowledge that is revealed now, overpowers the impressions in the seed. The seed holding many impressions with the ability to divide and multiply, is made infertile. When ṛtam is connected to the awareness, a new impression, born of the Samadhi erases all the impressions.

The practitioner gets established in the Knowledge, and becomes separate from the transient nature of this creation. There are no more associations. There is no past. He is born every moment, eternal.

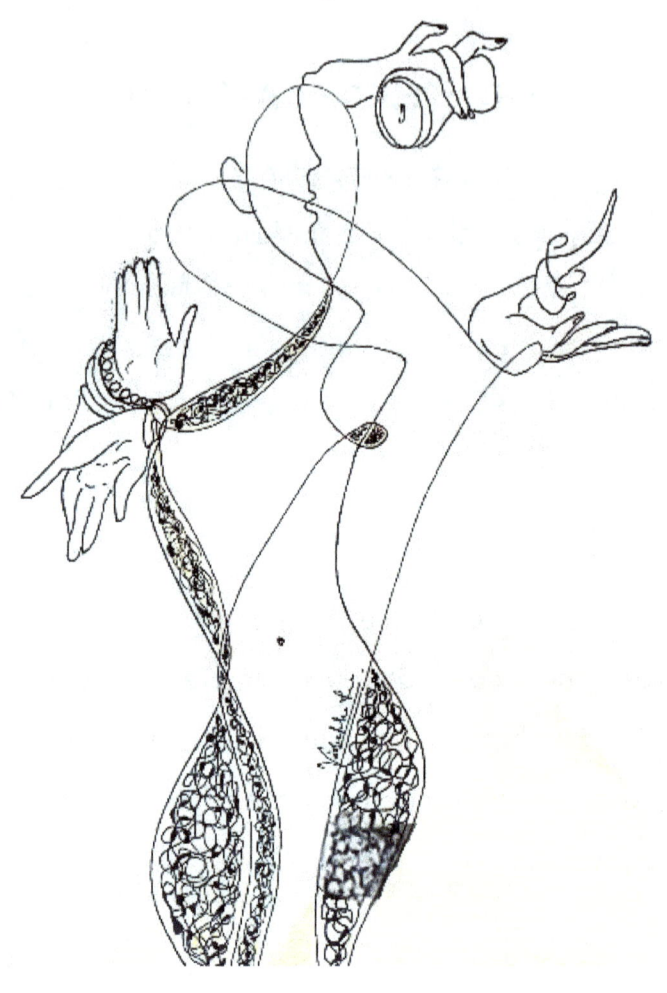

1.51

I AM

तस्यापि निरोधे सर्वनिरोधान्निर्बीजः समाधिः ॥
tasyāpi nirodhe sarvanirodhānnirbījaḥ samādhiḥ ॥
(tasyapi Nirodhe, sarva Nirodhan, nir-bija Samadhi)

When this impression is also dropped, Nirbijah Samadhi happens.

Where there is knowledge of God, the impression of the knowledge destroys all other impressions. When the knowledge, the truth is also dropped, dissolution, Liberation happens.

From knowing the cause of creation, one realizes one's own self to be the cause of creation, the creation itself, and its end. There is nothing but "I." One has realized the Self.

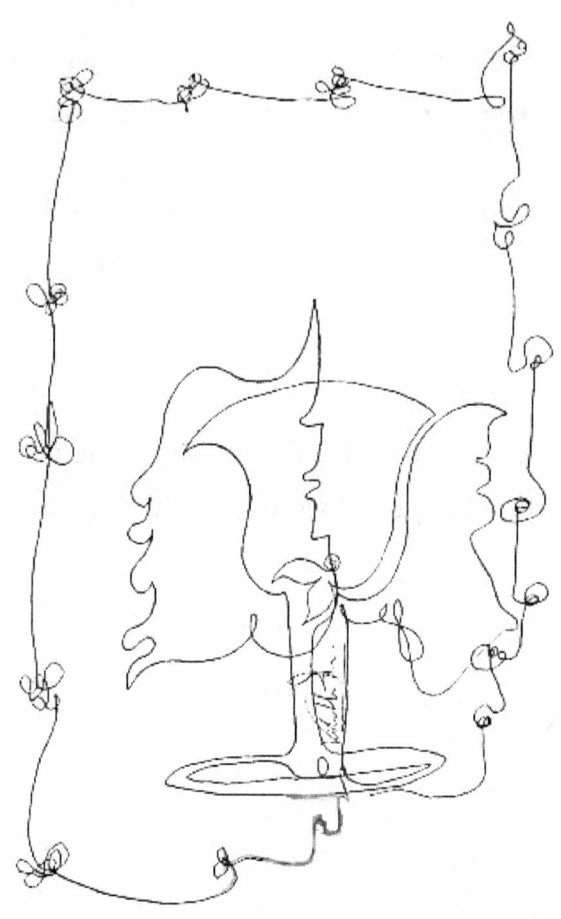

EPILOGUE

The realms of consciousness are mysterious, for they rest in non-doing. No knowledge can teach anyone about the secrets of the mind. It can only hope to give a tool and motivation for someone to start their journey on this path.

It is easy to forget the simple things, even on the spiritual path. Kindness and compassion carry unadulterated power. Humility and humor lighten the greatest of burdens. Playfulness achieves unmatched maturity. Therefore, not getting stuck in the intricacies of the technique, but moving ahead with faith, discipline, and playfulness will make sure we are stable in both means and the end.

सर्वे भवन्तु सुखिनः । सर्वे सन्तु निरामयाः ।
सर्वे भद्राणि पश्यन्तु । मा कश्चिद् दुःख भाग् भवेत् ॥
ॐ शान्तिः शान्तिः शान्तिः ॥

When faith has blossomed in life, Every step is led by the Divine.
Sri Sri Ravi Shankar

Om Namah Shivaya

जय गुरुदेव

ABOUT THE AUTHOR

A yoga-teacher, acupressure therapist, writer and poet, Dipanshu wears many hats. He graduated in B.E. Electronics and Communications, before doing his masters in Yogic Sciences. He founded ARNAVH YOGA in 2021, which aims to teach Yoga along with its values, in its traditional form. He is also the External Academic Expert - Center of Excellence (COE) – Yogic Studies, Woxsen University, Hyderabad. He has been teaching Yoga since 2020, and is currently undergoing training in Biodynamic Cranio-Sacral Therapy with Body Intelligence. He lives in Patiala, India with his family.

ABOUT THE ILLUSTRATOR

Vishakha holds a Master's degree in Yogic Science and Graduated in Fashion Communication Design, 200Hrs TTC from Yoga Alliance US, 100Hrs Aerial Yoga YACEP & YCB Level III Certified Evaluator, Educator & Trainer. An active member of Indian Yoga Association (IYA) and Yoga Alliance (YA) US. Vishakha often calls herself a Creative Yogi. In addition, she has over 700 hours of teaching experience in Yoga, with specialization in Mantra Chanting, Meditation, Vinyasa Flow, Ashtanga Vinyasa & Shivananda Flow.

Vishakha is currently an Assistant Professor in Design at Woxsen University, Hyderabad. She also serves as the Co-Chairperson of Center of Excellence (COE) – Yogic Studies at the institute, and Co Founder ARNAVH YOGA.

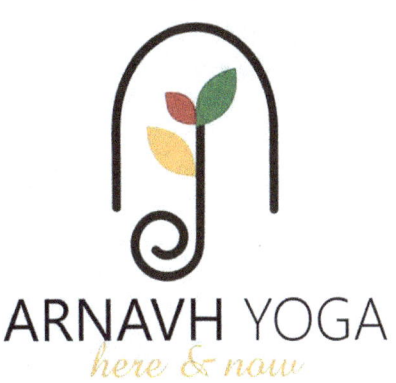

ARNAVH YOGA
here & now

Yoga is a way of life, a science of living, and a philosophy which answers questions that have scratched the minds of our race since we evolved a higher awareness. Yoga is ancient - probably older than Time (if that makes sense) as it deals with Time, Space, Matter and beyond.

ARNAVH is an attempt to make YOGA available and accessible to one and all. While the knowledge is ancient, our effort is to present Yoga that can be applied in the current times.

"We cannot teach you anything, for true knowledge is not gained, but realized. We are here to do Yoga with you - to share and build together a magnificent world. Simply put, we wish to be a reliable companion to your journey to health, joy and bliss."

https://www.arnavh.com/

https://www.instagram.com/arnavh_yoga/

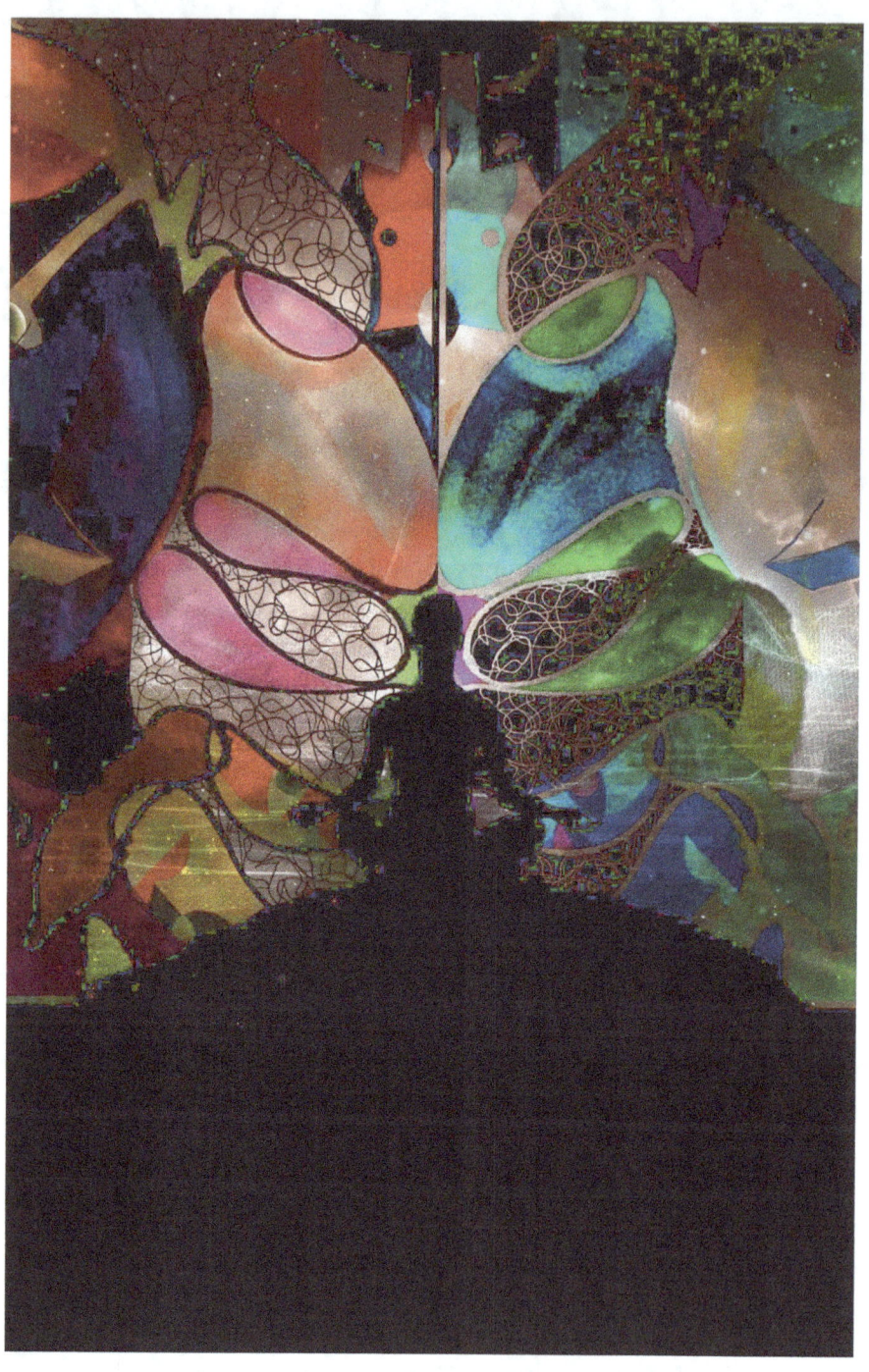

www.ingramcontent.com/pod-product-compliance
Lightning Source LLC
LaVergne TN
LVHW020427070526
838199LV00004B/307

1.46

THE SEED OF EXISTENCE

ता एव सबीजः समाधिः ॥
tā eva sabījaḥ samādhiḥ ॥
(Taa eva sa-Bija Samadhi)

These all are Samadhi with seed.

We are creations of our environment. We do not have any control over where we are born – the socio-economic status of the family and the country we are born in, domestic environment, availability of nutrition, emotional availability, and much more. Similarly, as we continue to grow from childhood, into adolescence and adulthood, we do not have control over the situations and circumstances that we encounter.

In Nature everything is balanced. Every organism must go through the cycle of birth, life, death, and repeat, but for human beings, life is a potential opportunity to get out of the cycle – like a seed has the potential to become a tree. But it needs to settle all its score. Nature always pays its debts.

The transactions yet to be completed are stored as impressions and travel lifetimes if they are resolved. These impressions are stored as if in a seed, and according to the intensity of life, many transactions surface as situations and people in our life to be resolved. The impressions, have the potential to express. If we live fully, without getting stuck in the game of doership and blame, then the seed burst and it empties itself, and when the body drops, there is nothing left for the consciousness to rid of, and there is dissolution.

It is not, however, necessary to go through all the transactions in the physical realm. Samadhi offers subtler realms where these impressions can be rid of in a fraction of time compared to the physical realm. All the states of samadhis discussed until now (Savitarka, Nirvitarka, Savichara, Nirvichara) do not access the subtle realm where this seed of impressions can be resolved. Hence, these Samadhis are called Sabija Samadhi – Samadhis with seed.

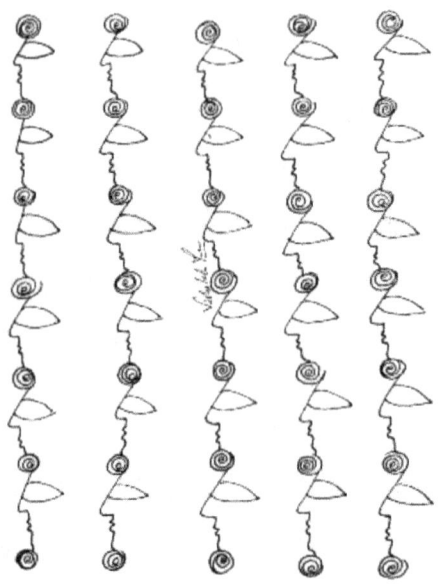